Living with Diabetes

Living with Diabetes

Heather Maclean and Barbara Oram

UNIVERSITY OF TORONTO PRESS

Toronto Buffalo London

© University of Toronto Press 1988
Toronto Buffalo London
Printed in Canada

ISBN 0-8020-6693-3

Canadian Cataloguing in Publication Data

Maclean, Heather.
   Living with diabetes

   ISBN 0-8020-6693-3

   1. Diabetes – Patients – Ontario – Toronto.
   2. Diabetes – Psychological aspects.
   I. Oram, Barbara, 1953-   . II. Title.

   RC660.M24 1988   616.4'62   C87-095204-8

Overview on pages 59–60, Option B's on pages 64–5, and
People at Work on page 89 adapted from *The Three Boxes of Life*
by Richard Bolles.
Copyright © 1981.
Used with permission of Ten Speed Press,
Box 7123, Berkeley, CA 94707, USA.

Contents

CHAPTER FIVE

CHAPTER SIX

CHAPTER SEVEN

CHAPTER EIGHT

CHAPTER NINE

Preface

This book was made possible through a grant from the Health Promotion Directorate of Health and Welfare Canada. The grant enabled us to extensively interview fifty adults who have diabetes. None of these people had developed any of the chronic complications of diabetes to the extent that their activity was seriously hampered. All of them lived in Metropolitan Toronto. We selected thirty-two people with insulin-dependent diabetes and eighteen with non-insulin-dependent diabetes. We had a balanced representation in the age ranges (from twenty to seventy-six) and gender (half men and half women). There was also a balanced representation according to the length of time since people developed diabetes. Twenty-one people had had diabetes for five years or less at the time of the interviews. Half of these had had it less than two years. We interviewed people until they felt they had told us all they could about what it is like to live with diabetes. On average, we talked to each individual three times. We tape-recorded and transcribed the conversations and through analysis identified the issues that were central to life with diabetes.

This book, which combines a narrative presentation with self-help exercises, presents these issues. Through the combination of descriptive narrative and an extensive use of actual quotes, the reader is acquainted with the issues that participants identified and the reactions they had. The narrative is an accurate representation of the frequency and intensity of the issues. The issues selected for presentation are those that reflected the concerns of many of our group. Although quotations have sometimes been abridged or slightly altered to fit the flow and maintain some semblance of brevity, we have always retained the spirit of the speaker. We have chosen pseudonyms to protect the confidentiality of the people we interviewed.

We wrote the book because we believe that the practical, everyday experiences of our participants are an important resource for helping other people with diabetes. There are very few books available which present the personal perspective of life with diabetes. Yet the people who have diabetes are the most knowledgeable about its stresses and strains and about the ways to manage it successfully. Because we interviewed a wide range of people we assume that most readers will be able to identify aspects of their own experiences in the accounts of others. This might help some feel less isolated. It might also help those who are searching for the words to describe their own thoughts and feelings and the reasons underlying their actions. Some may discover new ways of dealing with diabetes. Others may learn how various aspects of life, such as working conditions or family and friends, can influence the quality of one's life with diabetes.

Our assumption is that people will begin to question how the issues associated with diabetes that have been identified by others apply to their own lives. The exercises are designed to encourage this process. They are intended to help people who want to gain a deeper understanding of their reactions to diabetes and assess how their experiences are influenced by the people they know and the environment in which they live. Another purpose of the exercises is to help people who want to solve specific problems or who are generally dissatisfied with the impact of diabetes on their lives. Identifying and examining one's attitudes and feelings about a situation are an important first step toward effective change.

These are our reasons for writing this book. They are based on the perspective of diabetes as a complex condition which usually requires significant changes in people's everyday lives, changes which can be intrusive and demanding. This book is intended to help people who are trying to integrate these changes into their lives without seriously compromising their values and beliefs and the quality of their lives.

Those who are successfully coping with diabetes come to this book armed with a wealth of experience and a variety of learning needs. We invite them to explore the book and decide how it might be useful to them.

Although this book was written primarily for people who have diabetes and for their families, we hope that health professionals will also read this book, as it will provide them with the opportunity to walk in the shoes of their clients. Furthermore, the issues addressed in the book can serve as a focus for discussion about potential difficulties that clients may encounter. We hope, too, that the exercises will be useful to people who teach in diabetes education programs. The exercises can be assigned as homework or used with a small group format to encourage discussion about the personal aspects of integrating diabetes into one's life.

Acknowledgments

There are many people who contributed to the development of this book and who deserve a sincere thank you. First and foremost, this book rests on the willingness of all the participants in the study to generously share their experiences and viewpoints. This book tells their stories.

I would like to acknowledge the contribution of Barbara Oram, the co-author of this book. Barbara worked on the proposal to research and write this book and helped obtain funding. She was employed as project director and played a crucial role in the project management which included significant phases of data collection and analysis. She contributed to the first draft of chapters 3 through 7, including the exercises, and contributed to the revisions of the fourth and final draft of the manuscript. Barbara would like to recognize the contribution of Robert Snell, whose demonstration of the practical, everyday aspects of life with diabetes had a strong influence on the way she formulated her interest in the topic and her work on the project.

Sandy Samuels and Sarah Wales Marko, along with Barbara, conducted the interviews. Their skilful listening and questioning and their respect for the unique experiences of each participant added to the quality of the interviews. Sandra Horney, a graduate student, worked as a part-time xii Acknowledgments

research assistant on this project and contributed to the initial drafting of two chapters. Don Maudsley offered supportive criticism and played a major role in the development of the exercise portions of the book. Sue Ferrier and Charles Kahn both contributed their editorial assistance and Sue provided much-needed logistical help. Thank you also to Cheri Hernandez and Mike McFarland for their help and support in the early stages of the project and Heather Ramsey at the Health Promotion Directorate, Ontario Region, Health and Welfare Canada, for her constructive criticism. Finally, I gratefully acknowledge the advice, assistance, and support provided by the members of the Publications Committee and the Public Relations Department of the Canadian Diabetes Association. We are delighted to be able to produce this book in conjunction with this Association.

This project received a contribution from the Health Promotion Directorate, Health and Welfare Canada. The views expressed herein are solely those of the authors, and do not necessarily represent the official policy of the Department of National Health and Welfare.

H.M., September 1987

Living with Diabetes

CHAPTER ONE

The path to learning

The prospect of dealing with a chronic disease for the rest of one's life is not a welcome one. But the majority of people we interviewed learned to master it and lead full, productive lives. This book is a description of the issues that were central to their lives with diabetes. We hope that reading about their experiences will help you better understand aspects of your own life in relation to having diabetes as well as provide ideas for those of you who would like to more effectively deal with this often demanding condition.

We are directing the book primarily to those of you who have diabetes. However, we also believe that coping with diabetes requires help. It requires partnerships with family and friends, with health professionals, with diabetes organizations, and with other individuals and groups interested in enhancing the quality of life for people facing a lifelong chronic condition. So we hope that these partners will read this book, too. It will help them better understand what the daily challenge of living with diabetes is about.

The book is divided into ten chapters. This first chapter introduces the book and describes the learning theory on which this book is based. You may be able to identify the way(s) in which you tend to learn in the various approaches to learning described. Chapter 2 presents a brief overview of the condition. The following chapters trace the sequence from the diagnosis of diabetes, through to issues such as learning more about it, help and support, impact on relationships, the role of family and friends, and finally the ultimate goal of all participants – balance and control. It ends with a summary of the host of feelings generated by living with a chronic illness.

Most chapters are organized into two sections. The first section consists of a narrative that outlines what our participants thought were the important features of learning to live with diabetes. The issues they discussed are frequently illustrated with direct quotations. These quotes communicate better than we ever can what it feels like to confront diabetes. The second section contains a series of exercises to help you think about your own situation and to see if the ideas and concerns presented in the narrative apply to you. They are designed to help you gain insight into your experience and to sort out the steps you can take to set diabetes in perspective. Some exercises are designed to be done on your own. Some work better when done in a group where you have others to stimulate your thinking and share ideas. We make suggestions about how to use the exercises, but you may want to make some changes. You might choose to disregard parts of them, or invent new ones. They are intended to trigger your thinking and you are the best judge of what might do that. On the other hand, you might not be familiar with self-help exercises and be tempted to ignore them. We encourage you to try them. Reserve some quiet time, find a comfortable place, a pen and paper, and treat yourself to the opportunity to assess where you are with diabetes and where you would like to be. Look at the time spent as an investment in your health and well-being.

The central belief on which this book is founded is that people's everyday experiences are an important resource for learning. Your experiences and those of others with diabetes are valuable sources of knowledge that are often overlooked and undervalued. The narrative and exercises are presented to help you learn from what our participants experienced as well as from your own experiences of having diabetes.

How do we learn?

Many of us think of learning as something that only happens in a classroom or when a teacher is present. We all know the expression 'experience is the best teacher,' yet we often forget that, as adults, much of our learning comes informally through our day-to-day experience. This is also true with diabetes. There is a lot to learn through classes, reading, and/or one-on-one teaching by a health professional. But it is only through putting these facts and ideas into action that you can assess how they fit with your values, beliefs, and everyday practices and determine the adjustments that feel comfortable to you. This is a long and often continuous process of learning which might involve such things as trying out new behaviours as well as examining and sometimes redefining your attitudes and emotions in an effort to find a balance between your personal needs and those associated with the management of diabetes.

A model of learning

David Kolb, an expert on learning, has suggested that people learn using four different activities: experiencing, reflecting, building idea frameworks, and testing out new behaviours. Generally the learning process or cycle encompasses all four activities. The cycle looks like this:

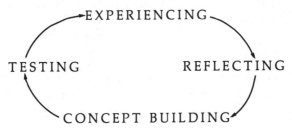

When we learn we can start anywhere on the cycle. Most of us have a preference for one or two of these activities and emphasize them over the others. By expanding our use of the less preferred activities we might find that we learn more easily, faster, and with more enjoyment. We are using this model, known as the Experiential Learning Model, because we think it is similar to the learning processes described by the people we interviewed. Here is a brief description of each activity in the model.

Experiencing

We jump into a situation and see how it feels, what is involved, and what has to be done. It is like a process of trial and error. With diabetes, many people, following diagnosis, need some time just living with it day by day. This way they develop a sense of what it will mean for them. Without this concrete experiencing, diabetes does not feel real. For example, you can read about adjusting your insulin to compensate for exercise but you need to experience first hand, how exercise affects your blood sugar before you know what this adjustment is all about.

Reflecting

We look back at our experiences and examine our feelings about them to try and understand more clearly what is happening to us and what it means for how we would like to change. When we reflect we ponder or contemplate. When you go to a party and overindulge in food or alcohol you might reflect on it the next day. You might review what you did. You might ask yourself how you felt about it. You might think about the things that contributed to your behaviour and examine what you could have done differently. This process is reflection.

Building idea frameworks

Building idea frameworks is a phrase used to describe how we understand information by labelling ideas in a systematic way so they make sense to us. Sometimes we do this labelling ourselves, often as an end product of reflection. Sometimes it is done for us by others. This happens when we read a book, listen to a lecture, or watch a TV program on a specific topic. The author, teacher, or producer tries to present material in such a way that it will be easy to learn because the ideas 'make sense.' A class on the diabetes diet will consist of an idea framework that will help you understand the reasons for the diet and provide tips on how to follow it. Thus you will learn key ideas: carbohydrates and blood sugar, food groups, measuring, timing of meals, etc. This is an idea framework.

Testing

When we test something out we take an idea or an activity and we try it out in a real situation. We experiment with something in order to learn more about it and to see if it brings the results we want. You might experiment with different doses of insulin prior to heavy exercise to see which dose is most appropriate. Or you might try out some different behaviours the next time you go to a party. For example, you might decide to drink wine instead of hard liquor or take only a half portion of dessert and see if you feel better about your behaviour.

These descriptions illustrate how we learn using the four activities of the Experiential Learning Model. Sometimes we learn using only one activity, but sometimes we use all four activities and learn in a cyclical way. We experience a situation, think about it, develop labels or ideas to describe what happened, and then decide to try a different approach. Then we move through the cycle again until we are satisfied with what we have learned. When we are satisfied, we feel as if we have integrated something new into our lives. This process can happen quickly or slowly. Occasionally we learn something with a great 'aha.' More often, it takes us months or years. Adjusting to diabetes can take a long time. There are a lot of little learnings along the way, but most of our study participants found it took a long time to feel that they had comfortably integrated it into their lives. However, even this sense of integration did not signify an end to learning about diabetes. New life circumstances emerged as did new learning needs. But, having once accomplished a major victory over diabetes, they now found it easier to meet the new challenges with optimism.

The narrative sections of each chapter contain many examples of how the people we interviewed learned about the practical side of life with diabetes using parts or all of the activities in this learning model. The actual narrative itself is an example of an idea framework. We have culled from our interviews the basic ideas that we think portray the central issues that people faced in coping with diabetes. We present these ideas in an organized way so you can learn, from this idea framework, what others experienced. It might also help you find 'labels' to describe what you are facing and help you learn about yourself.

The exercise sections of the chapters are designed to help you expand your repertoire of learning activities – to try out all four phases of the Experiential Learning Model. The exercises usually begin by asking you to reflect on and assess your own experience. Activities such as diary- or journal-writing, sentence completions, and scenario-writing are geared to helping you relive the actual events and bring back information that may have escaped your notice earlier. Questions that probe feelings around specific events invite you to identify these feelings and to explore them. Often this activity helps you better understand your feelings and to reassess your situation. Suggestions are included to help you design and experiment with new courses of action for new coping strategies and behaviour changes.

The exercises encourage you to outline a number of ways to meet the goals you have identified. One course of action you try might not work. It may be that you are trying to change something over which you do not have a lot of control. Unfortunately, we cannot control all the people and aspects of our environment which influence our daily lives. For example, it would be a difficult task as an individual to develop a diabetes education program in your community. Yet if you could form or join a group of people working towards this goal it might be achievable. One of the goals of the Canadian Diabetes Association is to be an advocate to governments, business, and the general public on behalf of all people affected by diabetes in order to increase awareness and influence and effect positive changes in attitudes, policies, and practices. The ultimate goal we would all like to achieve is to find the cure for diabetes. None of us has the power to do this alone, yet there are many dedicated people who are working collectively to try to make this discovery.

Sometimes we learn things on our own and sometimes we learn with other people. Learning with others can be helpful because we have a sounding board – someone who will listen and help us clarify ideas. When others present their viewpoints they might trigger new learnings for us. There are a number of ways in which people with diabetes can learn with others. Later in this book you will read about diabetes education classes sponsored by many hospitals across the country. These classes frequently include group discussion and problem-solving sessions. Local branches of the Canadian Diabetes Association offer services such as classes on specific topics and may sponsor peer support groups where the primary purpose is to provide a forum for people with diabetes to meet others in the same situation. Sessions with health professionals provide another opportunity to learn about coping with diabetes. Many people spoke highly of health professionals who expressed interest and concern about their welfare. These professionals took time to both ask and answer questions and to help identify strategies to manage diabetes. Don't forget that they, too, learn from these discussions and in turn pass their insights on to others. There are less obvious ways to learn with others. You could consider becoming part of a 'buddy system' with a person with diabetes who has more experience than you. You could search for a pen pal. Newsletters of local diabetes associations will print letters from people looking for ways to meet others. You can use many of the exercises in this book as a basis for discussion and further learning in any of these group settings.

Alternatively, you might prefer to learn on your own. In this case you will probably want to read a lot. (Later in the book we suggest other books to read.) You might wish to purchase a notebook to use with this book. In it you can jot down your reactions to what you read, try out the exercises, and perhaps make plans for changes you would like to make.

This book is not intended to be read in a single sitting or even in strict chapter sequence. It is meant to help you think about the significance of diabetes as a part of your life. This process will take time. Learning to live with diabetes is like embarking on a journey along a meandering road. It is not the destination but the actual journey that is important. The path is rarely straight or the ground level, and there are often unexpected diversions along the route. This book is a guidebook to help you negotiate the journey. Guidebooks describe routes that others have found. They suggest alternative courses and provide information on some of the sights along the way. They are not, however, prescriptions for travel. The joy of travelling is in charting your own course, encountering challenges, and learning and thriving in unfamiliar territory. We wish you *bon voyage*.

CHAPTER TWO

What is diabetes?

Diabetes is a chronic disorder that can strike at any stage of life. It can be controlled, but there is no known cure. Diabetes is not a single disorder but a group of disorders, all of which are characterized by glucose intolerance.

When the body breaks down carbohydrates from food it turns them into glucose, which is a type of sugar. Glucose is carried through the body by the blood and then enters into the body's cells, where it is used as a source of energy. Glucose needs insulin, a hormone produced by the pancreas, in order to get into the cells. The pancreas releases different amounts of insulin depending upon the amount and type of food eaten. In diabetes the body either a) does not produce any insulin or b) produces insufficient amounts of insulin or c) cannot use the available insulin properly.

Types of diabetes

There are four categories of disorders that are labelled diabetes mellitus. They are:

1 Type I or insulin-dependent diabetes (IDDM)

This type can develop at any age but is most common in those under thirty. Generally, these people do not produce any insulin and require injected insulin to sustain life. If insulin is not provided a condition called ketoacidosis develops. The extremely high blood-glucose levels allow poisonous substances called ketoacids to accumulate and these can cause death. Type I diabetes is believed to be an autoimmune disease. Because something is wrong with the body's immune system the cells in the pancreas that produce insulin are destroyed, thus necessitating insulin from an external source.

2 Type II or non-insulin-dependent diabetes (NIDDM)

The majority of people with Type II diabetes are over forty, although they, too, can develop it at any age. These people rarely totally lack insulin. The problem in Type II does not appear to be the destruction of the cells that produce insulin. Instead, it seems that the body cannot use the insulin in the way it is supposed to. Therefore, people with Type II diabetes are described as insulin resistant. Insulin therapy is occasionally required but in many cases the diabetes can be controlled by diet and weight loss. Sometimes pills (known as oral hypoglycemic agents) are used to treat this condition. Up to 80 per cent of people with Type II diabetes are obese and this is probably a factor in the development of the condition. The 20 per cent who are non-obese are more likely to require insulin therapy eventually.

3 Secondary diabetes

This type of diabetes develops as a side effect of other conditions, e.g. pancreatic disease, other endocrine diseases, or the administration of certain drugs.

4 Gestational diabetes

In this instance the diabetes develops with the onset of pregnancy because of the complex metabolic and hormonal changes. Although it disappears after delivery, these individuals are at a high risk of developing diabetes later in life.

Prevalence

Type I and Type II diabetes are, by far, the more common types. It has been estimated that over one million Canadians have diabetes, although half of them do not know they have it. Ninety to ninety-five per cent of all people with diabetes have Type II. The prevalence of diabetes increases with age. By age seventy, 10 per cent of the population has the condition.

Certain ethnic groups are more likely to develop diabetes, especially Blacks, North American Indians, and Mexicans. About 25 per cent of people with Type II diabetes have a family history of the condition. People who are overweight are far more likely to develop diabetes. The more overweight a person is the higher the risk becomes. Even a person who is only twenty to thirty pounds overweight triples his or her chances of developing Type II diabetes.

Only 5 to 10 per cent of the total population of people with diabetes have Type I. Type I used to be referred to as juvenile onset diabetes because it frequently develops during childhood or adolescence. Nonetheless, the chances of a child developing diabetes are small. Only thirteen out of ten thousand have developed it by age sixteen. Family history plays a role in the development of Type I diabetes, but it is less prominent than for Type II. If one parent has Type I diabetes the risk that his or her child will develop it is only 2 to 5 per cent.

Symptoms

The onset of symptoms is generally different in Type I and Type II diabetes. In Type I diabetes the symptoms often emerge abruptly and can be severe. The symptoms include extreme thirst, frequent urination, weight loss, and fatigue. Similar symptoms may occur, but in a milder form, in Type II diabetes. Frequently, though, there are no symptoms at all and the condition is discovered at the time of a routine medical examination.

There are a number of complications that may develop over time as a result of diabetes. The frequency of complications, the age of onset, and the intensity of the symptoms are unpredictable. They can vary in severity from insignificant to being so fully developed that a person can be continuously incapacitated. It is generally believed that individuals who keep their blood glucose levels as close as possible to those of people without diabetes may develop fewer complications. However, there is a lot of controversy about this issue in medical circles, and doctors voice strong opinions both for and against the importance of *rigid* maintenance of normal blood glucose levels. Other factors such as genes, hormones, and the environment appear to modify the progress and severity of the condition, but their roles are poorly understood. A great deal of current diabetes research is directed toward determining the relationship between blood glucose levels and the development of complications.

There are three major categories of complications. The first category involves the progressive thickening or damaging of the blood vessels, particularly in the eyes and the kidneys. Secondly, diabetes accentuates problems associated with cardiovascular disease including heart disease, hypertension, and strokes. Thirdly, people with diabetes can develop neuropathy, which can lead to a loss of sensation in the body extremities and to impotence. The potential impact of these complications is staggering and is a strong motivator to find a cure for diabetes. In the meantime a primary goal of the medical management of diabetes is to normalize blood glucose levels with the hope that this action will lower the risk of developing complications.

Diabetes management

Diabetes management includes diet, medication, and exercise. These forms of treatment are sufficiently complex that a considerable amount of education is necessary to help people integrate the management approaches into their day-to-day lives.

The diabetes diet is an integral part of treatment of both Type I and Type II diabetes. The diet is restricted in simple carbohydrates and animal fats. It must be eaten at regular intervals during the day, and must contain a prescribed amount of protein, carbohydrate and fat. Diets for people with Type II diabetes who are overweight are restricted in calories as well, because weight loss decreases the body's resistance to the insulin it produces.

The medication varies depending on the type of diabetes. People with Type I diabetes do not produce their own insulin. They must inject themselves with insulin one or more times a day to compensate for this deficiency. Many people with Type II diabetes do not need medication. Weight loss and the diabetes diet can together keep the condition under control. When this combination is not enough, pills, known as oral hypoglycemics, are given. These pills stimulate the pancreas to produce more insulin and help the body cells use up the glucose in the blood stream.

Regular physical exercise improves the effectiveness of both the diet and medication. It can lower both blood sugar and blood fats. Because of its impact on blood glucose it is necessary to coordinate exercise with medication.

Diabetes education is essential for good diabetes management. The diabetes health care team usually consists of physicians, nurses, dietitians, and social workers. All of these professionals help people learn about the various facets of management in one-to-one teaching and in classes. There are also many good books written to help people learn more about the whys and hows of diabetes management. In contrast, this book discusses diabetes from a personal, nonmedical viewpoint. We present our participants' experiences of living with diabetes in their communities as a valuable source of knowledge for others. We hope that this will provide you with some insight into your own thoughts, feelings, and actions in relation to diabetes and help those of you who would like to make some changes as a result. The remaining chapters of this book will lead you down the paths that others with diabetes have travelled and will provide guideposts, in the form of exercises, to help you find your way. The journey begins at diagnosis, the subject of the next chapter.

CHAPTER THREE

Diagnosis

Introduction

The initial period following the diagnosis of diabetes is traumatic for almost everyone who develops diabetes. The people we spoke with had vivid memories of the time leading up to and following the diagnosis. They described the events and their feelings as if they had occurred just recently. In this chapter we will recount the experiences of seven people. The stories we selected reflect a range of responses to the diagnosis. Some people accepted the diagnosis easily; others were extremely upset. Of the seven, four were dependent on insulin injections. Tim, who was nineteen when he was diagnosed found diabetes very hard to accept. Craig, who was in his mid twenties, accepted it quite quickly and got on with his life. Gary, in his late thirties, was not surprised by the diagnosis. He knew his risks were high because his mother had diabetes. Gwyn, who was sixty-three, reacted with shock and anger. The three people who had non-insulin-dependent diabetes had reactions similar to insulin-dependent people even though this form of diabetes is considered less serious by the medical profession. The vignettes that follow all illustrate 1) the range of symptoms prior to diagnosis, 2) the reactions people had to learning they had diabetes, and 3) the experiences they had as they began to adjust to the fact that diabetes was with them for life.

Insulin-dependent diabetes

Tim

Tim was nineteen years old when he developed diabetes. Eight years later, his recollections were still vivid. Tim had recently finished high school and had just passed the three-month probationary period on his first job. At the age of nineteen, he felt that life was 'shaping up.' He was making money and could contribute to the family by paying board at home. He had many friends and led a busy life. It was November, and the hockey season was well under way. Tim loved sports and since childhood had always played tennis, baseball, and road hockey. Because he believed his health was important, he chose not to smoke or drink excessively, although many of his friends did both. It was very frustrating, then, when he began to feel sick. He described his symptoms:

I had been feeling really tired. I'd go play hockey and be exhausted after the game. I had been eating like a horse, yet had lost about thirty to forty pounds. I was very thin and weak. People would come up to me and say, 'Tim, you're not looking well!'

Tim's doctor gave him a thorough medical examination. The following day he received a call from the doctor's office asking him to take a cab to the hospital immediately. The blood tests, which revealed an overactive thyroid, were so high that the doctor feared he might die.

Tim's stay in the hospital was very hard on him. He recalled what happened:

I was in very bad condition in the hospital. I had lost more weight; I couldn't lift anything; I was deteriorating like nothing. They were taking all these blood tests to try to figure out how to treat the problem. I'll never forget what happened on the fourth day I was in the hospital. The nurse came into my room and took my chocolate cookies. I yelled at her and said, 'Don't you dare touch those, they're mine!' She argued that the doctor had instructed her to take all food away from me. I asked her why. She didn't tell me. She just took them away and said that the doctor would be in to talk to me. That just blew my mind. I knew what was wrong with me; I had an overactive thyroid. But I didn't know anything about it. I was in a really bad state.

That day the doctor told him he had diabetes but that they needed to take more blood tests to confirm their suspicion. Tim knew nothing about diabetes other than having previously heard the word. His main concern was why his food had been taken away. When told it was because of the diabetes, Tim was astonished: 'You've got to be kidding, I can't eat cookies because I have diabetes!'

Later that day the doctor confirmed the diagnosis. Tim recalled his nonchalant reaction. 'I thought it was a simple thing that could be cured with a pill, so I said, "Who cares, give me the pill and it'll go away." ' The next day he was given his first shot of insulin. They told him what they were doing but it was hard to grasp its significance:

The next morning they gave me a shot of insulin, but I didn't think anything of it because I had so many needles in the hospital. They gave me the needle for four or five days before they told me that I had to give it to myself. The nurse said, 'When you leave here, you will be on the needle for the rest of your life.' I said, 'You've got to be

*kidding!' She tried to tell me that the doctor had told me,
but he hadn't.*

*I thought, 'That's it. I can't do that.' I was terrified of
needles. I didn't want to take a needle. I thought I had to
take insulin while I was in the hospital because it would
cure me and get me out of the hospital. The nurse taught
me how to inject insulin, but I wasn't listening. I just
looked at her. I wasn't in a condition to learn anything! I
didn't know what was happening to me. I thought I was
on my deathbed.*

Tim refused to take the needle so the nurse brought the doctor in to persuade him to reconsider. He said, 'Tim, you are
going to have to take it. There are millions of people with diabetes out there that do it.' This information did not help con-
vince him because he saw himself as quite separate from
others with diabetes. In addition, he wanted to know what
would happen if he did not take insulin:

*I thought they were pulling my leg, trying to get me to
take the needle. They told me that I would last about
three, maybe four days. I would go into a coma and might
never come out. I said, 'Do you mean that if I don't take
the needle I'm going to die? Is it that serious?' I was completely depressed. That night I lay in bed trying to figure
out what was going on, what they were trying to tell me. I
didn't know what I was supposed to do. They had thrown
a diet at me and told me that I had to stick a needle in me,
and no more cookies – I was all mixed up.*

At the same time the dietitian arrived and explained the diet
to Tim and his mother. He could not understand why he had
to learn about the diet and was determined to continue eating
as he had before.

During those two weeks in hospital Tim was confused and

deeply disturbed by what was happening to him. Fortunately, his mother sensed his turmoil and knew what to say to lift his spirits. One night she phoned him:

She just asked how I was feeling. I told her that if I had a gun I would do myself in. That's how bad I was feeling. I broke down and told her, 'I can't handle this. There's no way. I can't do it.' She tried to calm me down. She told me that she had learned the diet and would help me along, but that I was going to have to do my part. I was so upset that I wasn't about to listen to anyone, not even my mother. I said to her, 'No way, I know I have diabetes and I just want to end it all now.' I had hit the low point. I talked to her for about an hour on the phone and she made me feel a bit better.

Because of the diet and the insulin Tim soon began to feel better, although it took a long time to recover his strength. He was off work for five to six months, an unusually long time period. The fact that he had diabetes still weighed heavily, but time passed and life slowly began to improve. His mother helped enormously, as did his friends. They called on him regularly and treated him no differently than they had prior to the diagnosis:

When I got out of the hospital, I was told that I would have to take it easy at first until I got my strength back. After a few months I started to play baseball with my friends. They would call on me and ask me if I wanted to come out and give it a try. They got me going. The guys were like an inspiration to me. They kept calling on me, and they kept me busy. The less time I sat around and thought about what had happened to me the better. It seemed like they didn't care; they just didn't treat me differently. It was amazing.

Tim's account of his diagnosis portrays the shock that accompanies the change from being active and healthy to being ill and helpless. His words reflect the anxiety he felt because of the shock, the confusion, and the uncertainty. We can see how his first response – denial – made it difficult for him to learn the knowledge and skills necessary to treat it. Initially he could not take diabetes seriously, but once the implications dawned on him he became very depressed. When the reaction to the diagnosis of diabetes is so powerful it is little wonder that it takes time to get back to normal. Tim needed a few months to get back on his feet and face life again, and support from others was an important factor in his recovery.

Craig

At the age of twenty-five Craig moved west to begin a new job. He had a wife, a young son, and another child on the way. His work demanded long hours and a lot of travelling; he had concluded that the pressures of the job must be getting to him:

I was feeling lousy. I started to lose weight and was having difficulty getting up in the morning. My wife was concerned. I went to the doctor, but he couldn't find anything wrong. I kept roaring right along until it reached ridiculous proportions. It crossed my mind that I might have a serious problem.

Craig dropped into his doctor's office one afternoon to have blood tests done because he was not feeling any better. He also had to drive a friend out to the airport and planned to return to the doctor's office on his way home. While waiting for the plane, Craig and his friend went for a drink. This friend was astonished at how much he drank in the short time they had to wait. Craig admitted that he did not know why he was so thirsty. On returning to the doctor's office he received a shock:

When I stepped off the elevator, the nurse grabbed me and said, 'The doctor wants to see you right away.' I walked past all the people in the waiting room into the doctor's office. I remember him literally dropping something when he saw me. 'You've got to get to the hospital as fast as you can,' he said. I was stunned. 'Why?' The doctor replied, 'Because you're a chronic diabetic. I can't believe that I overlooked the obvious symptoms the last time you were here. Your blood sugar level is astronomical!'

Craig can barely recall what happened after leaving the doctor's office. He remembered getting a friend to take him home because the doctor insisted that he was not well enough to drive. He checked into the hospital that afternoon and spent the long evening and night pondering what was happening to him:

Finding out I had diabetes was a shock to my system. There was a lot of confusion, a lot of questions that I was forced to deal with. It wasn't something that could be put off until I was feeling a little better about it. The first big concern was not knowing what diabetes was – what it meant. I had grand plans for the future and I could see them going down the toilet. I had some real fears about what was going to happen to me. Would my company still want me? Was I going to be able to get insurance? Was I looking at a complete and dramatic shift away from my life plans? I really felt diabetes was going to affect everything. It was screwing me right into the ground. I thought, 'If this is the ball game, then why even bother?' I understand now why a friend of mine with diabetes got

*himself totally drunk and hit a telephone pole. I can see it
happening. My thoughts were very negative and irrational,
but I had no reason to be rational at the time. I was in
shock for the first day.*

Craig's mind was 'racing away and thinking all kinds of
weird and frightening thoughts.' He decided to 'put the
brakes on' and 'spend a couple of weeks seeing what diabetes
was all about.' Once he had more information he could
decide how serious diabetes was. He promised himself that he
would be out of the hospital for Christmas and set about
meeting his goal.

One of the first things Craig learned in the hospital was
how to inject insulin:

*It was extremely difficult to do. No one in his right mind
inflicts pain on himself. I can remember sitting on the side
of the bed thinking that I had done all kinds of things
harder than this, but I still couldn't put that needle into
myself. For me there was a block. It was just like a
concrete wall. It's not very big and not supposed to be
painful yet I could not force my hand to do it. The nurses
overcame the situation by refusing to feed me until I
injected myself. I was faced with the choice of slight
discomfort from a self-inflicted wound or starving to death.
I just sat there and sat there. I eyed the breakfast they had
brought in and thought if I wait another five minutes those
eggs are going to get cold. I was starving. I eventually did
it, but it wasn't easy that first time.*

Craig also learned what an insulin reaction was like. 'I
think they wanted me to experience it. There's no greater
teacher than experience.' It happened quickly and was quite
frightening because he had no idea what was happening to
him.

Hoping to be discharged, Craig had a long discussion with his doctor on the day before Christmas. The doctor warned him that he could run into all kinds of problems and would have to make certain adjustments. Craig finally convinced the doctor to let him go by promising he would come back to the hospital if he could not manage. That was thirteen years ago. He has not had to be hospitalized for a diabetes-related problem since.

Craig recalled many things pertaining to how he coped through those first few months after leaving the hospital:

It was mind over matter. I had a lot of anxiety around not being able to do my job. It was fortunate that I had a good boss who was understanding. I remember coming out of the hospital and feeling a different sense of urgency than I had before. It was like I was going to run out of time because diabetes was going to shorten my life. My father had died relatively early in life, and I was of the opinion that longevity wasn't of any real importance as long as you accomplished something in the time you were given. I had hustled enough before but felt a different sense of urgency now. I was in a panic for the first year.

Craig's philosophy, inherited from his father, had always been that you have to do the best with what time you have in life. This philosophy helped quell his anxiety and strengthened his determination. His recovery time was much faster than Tim's. Almost immediately he made plans to bring diabetes under control and get on with his life. He was eager and able to learn what he could about managing effectively because of his increased sense of urgency to accomplish things in his life. In summing up how he intended to approach diabetes he said, 'I will roll with the punches and persist in all of the things I want to do.' As we will see later, Craig's life has been rich and full in spite of diabetes.

Gary

It was not a surprise to Gary when he developed diabetes at the age of thirty-seven. His mother had diabetes for over twenty-five years, and Gary was aware of its hereditary nature and the possibility that he might one day develop it as well.

Throughout the years of living with his mother, Gary made a point of learning about the condition. He had periodic blood and urine tests when he was in his teens and an annual check-up as an adult. One year his blood sugar was a little high, but by moderating his diet he brought it back to normal, and everything seemed fine. Then four years ago he was admitted to hospital with an attack of pancreatitis. These attacks had occurred over a ten-year period and frequently coincided with 'a rather prolific consumption of alcohol for several months.' At the time of his last attack he was told that his pancreas was sufficiently damaged that the attacks were now occurring spontaneously without alcohol. He had surgery to remove the damaged portion of his pancreas that November and slowly recuperated in December. When he went for a checkup, the doctor told him that he would be back to normal in another couple of months. Gary, however, felt concerned:

I found that I was tired, but I thought it was because of the surgery and the hectic pace at work. I was running a conference, and there was a fair amount of stress involved. I was also eating a lot and drinking fluids. At the meetings I went through a jug of water in the course of a morning. I was up during the night going to the washroom and drinking more fluids. This went on for a week and I thought, 'This is not normal.' In the back of my mind I was thinking that these symptoms sounded very familiar.

He decided to test his urine and discovered sugar. As he had an appointment with his surgeon the next day, he phoned and suggested that the doctor take a blood test. The test confirmed his suspicions – his blood sugar was so high that he was admitted to hospital.

In the hospital Gary read all he could about diabetes. He discovered that the diabetes could have been triggered by the trauma of the major surgery, especially because he lost a third of his pancreas.

After two weeks Gary's blood sugar level was stabilized, and he believed that in that period he came to accept the condition:

I had been psyching myself up for years that it might happen. Now I don't have to worry about when it is going to happen because it is here. I think that I might have felt some resentment toward my mother and questioned, 'Why me? Why not one of the other members of my family?' Apart from that I wasn't surprised. I took it in my stride. I really did.

Gary indicated that diabetes had been a cause for concern in his family. His mother, in particular, carried a burden of guilt. Gary described what happened when he told his family that he had developed diabetes:

I was fairly lighthearted about it. I told my sister that she didn't have to worry about getting it anymore because I got it now; I was the lucky one. My mother started to cry. She blamed herself and felt guilty. I told her there was nothing she could do about it and nothing I could do about it; that was the way it was.

In Gary's case the onset of diabetes was not unexpected. He seemed to believe that his own behaviour (excessive drinking) had played some role in the development of diabetes. His familiarity with the condition and how it was treated appeared to ease the adjustment process.

Gwyn

Six weeks before one Christmas Gwyn had been feeling the pressures of her work in a way that was unusual for her. She had always performed well under pressure and still did at the age of sixty-three:

I could come home after work at five thirty, sit down for ten minutes and relax, and be gone for the rest of the night until midnight, then go to bed and get up at six.

But this year it was different:

I could not seem to get at it. Even when the pressure was on I couldn't produce. I was finding it just a drag to get out of bed. I thought it was just that there was a lot of work to be done.

Other people had commented to her that she was not her usual, energetic self. She had been to the doctor for her annual checkup in October and concluded that if anything had been wrong he would have phoned her. Nonetheless, her behaviour was alarming:

Around the first of December I had a two o'clock meeting. I remember deliberately writing down something that happened at the first of the meeting. After that I don't know what went on. I slept through the meeting. When the meeting was finished, the committee members woke me up and jokingly told me I could leave now. I was literally falling asleep in meetings. It was just awful! I was frustrated. The

*afternoons were absolutely terrible. I had to get up and
walk around because I would fall asleep. People told me to
go to the doctor and get some energy pills or something.*

Over that Christmas Gwyn had time off. She had wanted
to do some cross-country skiing, but she just did not have the
energy. During the first week of January she drove downtown for an afternoon meeting. On her way home she had an
unsettling experience:

*I left downtown at about four o'clock. As I was driving, I
realized that for a flick of a second I had fallen asleep and
the car had gone just over the yellow line on the road. I
thought, 'What is the matter with me? If I'm this tired,
I better pull over and have a few winks.' I pulled into the
parking lot at 4:45 and woke up at 8:30. That really scared
me. I knew I had to find out where my energy had gone
because it was really getting me down. I phoned the doctor
that week and went in to see him.*

The doctor's initial reaction to Gwyn's complaint of fatigue
was to suggest that she was working too hard and needed a
holiday. Because of the pressures of work Gwyn did not feel
she could afford to take time off. The doctor sent her to the
lab for x-rays and blood tests. Later that day he phoned to
tell her she had diabetes. When asked if she had any history
of diabetes in the family, Gwyn suddenly remembered that
her mother had elevated blood sugars in the months before
she died. She also recalled that her older brother had developed diabetes late in life and had to stop driving because his
eyes had been affected by it.

Gwyn described her immediate reaction to the diagnosis:

*I was very upset. I didn't know how I was going to live
with diabetes. What I'd heard about it were horror stories.*

I didn't think I would be able to work or do anything. I remembered people saying that if you've got diabetes you can't do any sports activities, so I thought I wouldn't be able to go skiing. I'd have to watch what I ate. It would be a drag if I went out anywhere because I would have to tell people I couldn't have that because I have diabetes. I couldn't see how I could live any kind of normal existence at all. Yet, I wasn't willing to curtail my activities because of diabetes. It was really a controversy within myself.

She was filled with uncertainty:

Why would it be me rather than someone else? Where on earth did I pick this up? It was just a question mark. Why did my body run out and somebody else's kept running? I felt a lot of anger. Even though the doctor was reassuring, I didn't know what was happening to myself and wasn't quite ready to accept what he was telling me. I didn't know what I had done wrong. I didn't know what to do to get back on the right track again, even though the doctor explained the various ways of dealing with diabetes.

Her doctor gave Gwyn the choice of either going to the hospital for two weeks or attending a two-week diabetes-education program where she would learn about diabetes and how to cope with it. Gwyn opted for the education program. This helped her understand the condition and the treatment for it, but she was still upset:

In the pit of my stomach I was still saying, 'It's not for me.' I am a very independent person. The fact that I was going to have to be dependent on somebody or something for the rest of my life was a real infringement on my independence. I think that was really hard for me to accept. I didn't want to cope with illness. This wasn't like other ill-

*nesses I had experienced because it wasn't going to go
away. I was stuck on insulin for the rest of my life. It was
a real infringement on me as a human being.*

For Gwyn the first six months were difficult. She was
determined that diabetes was not going to interfere with her
life even though her diet was restricted. She had to begin to
educate her family and friends about diabetes, especially
about the foods she could eat.

Gwyn had a lot of questions. The reading she did told her
what not to do instead of what to do. The main message she
received was that she had to be careful – 'careful of this and
careful of that.' She described her confusion:

*I've got diabetes, what do I do? Where do I go? What do I
look for? I had a lot of questions that I somehow had to
get answered myself.*

Despite her confusion, Gwyn eventually learned what she
needed to know. In fact, her gloomy predictions were not
fulfilled:

*It's been easy enough to live with once I got over the initial
frustration and depression. It takes a lot of sorting out. I
belong to a community that would look after me if things
went wrong, so I didn't have to worry that way. I was
relatively scot-free of other pressures that can add to the
condition. I really had to look at it day by day at the
beginning. There may be a few days when I'm not going to
feel up to scratch, but I can cope with that if I take it a
day at a time. It took time to learn that.*

Non-insulin-dependent diabetes

Michael

The symptoms Michael had were familiar to him because his
father had diabetes. He had suspected that his thirst and

extreme fatigue might have been a sign that he, too, was developing it. On the other hand, his fatigue could have been a result of the demands of the new job he had started four months earlier. Three years before, at thirty-two, his blood sugar had been slightly elevated. He had been warned of his potential to inherit the condition. He knew that he should go to the doctor, but he kept postponing it even though his symptoms began to intrude on his life:

For about six months I was feeling tired all the time. I wouldn't notice it if I kept busy, but as soon as I sat down in front of the television and relaxed I would drop off to sleep. It caused a lot of friction between my wife and me. I wasn't interested in her. I was totally bored at home. All I wanted to do was sleep. My mind started to blank out, and I was falling asleep at seven o'clock at night.

Finally, Michael was forced to go to a doctor because of his employer's policy that management staff have a medical checkup every year. A blood test confirmed his suspicions about diabetes. Michael recalled how he felt:

It was comforting to find out that there was a physical cause instead of a mental cause for the way I had been feeling for the last six months and that something could be done about it. My wife was relieved as well. Even though I had thought about having diabetes I was aware that there might be other reasons for the symptoms.

Michael described his father's reaction when he told him he had diabetes:

He started lecturing me on what he had done wrong. He hadn't paid attention to anything. He had a stroke in December. My father was the epitome of what can go wrong if you're a diabetic.

Michael's wife also had a strong reaction:

She thought I was going to die within a week. Shortly after I found out I had diabetes, I went out and planted new flower beds in the garden. She thought I was totally over-doing it. I was sick and should not be going out and doing these things. She was overly concerned, which became irritating after a while.

Michael identified a number of factors that helped him accept diabetes. He was reassured by the fact that he had friends who had developed diabetes as teenagers but now seemed unaffected by it. He also found help through reading extensively about diabetes and by attending a diabetes-education program. There Michael met people who had developed some of the complications of diabetes. 'I saw what I didn't want to become. It motivated me to do something about diabetes.'

Michael had been overweight for most of his life, but he lost thirty-five pounds soon after he was diagnosed. It was important to see progress. Weighing in at the doctor's office once a week became a source of motivation. The drop in blood sugar as he lost weight was another incentive to keep trying. Best of all, he was feeling better. His philosophy of life also helped him in those first months after diagnosis:

I live one day at a time. I don't worry about what's going to come tomorrow and I don't care what happened yesterday. All I really care about is surviving today.

John

When John was forty-five, he found out during a routine annual checkup that he had diabetes. It was a totally unex-pected occurrence, and the experience, even after twenty years, was clearly etched in his mind:

I went for a routine check-up. Like most people I took it for granted everything was going to be okay. When I found out I had diabetes, I was shocked and frightened. It came like a bolt out of the sky.

Prior to diagnosis, diabetes was merely a word to him. He knew nothing about it except that 'it meant having to shoot yourself with a needle every day.' He was afraid of the unknown, but some of his fear was alleviated when told that he could control diabetes by taking a pill. As he learned more about it, he became aware of the difference it would make in his life. One of the first things he realized was that he had to make changes in his eating habits:

All of a sudden I had to follow a controlled diet. I loved sweets. I'd sit down and have a sundae for breakfast at work. I felt deprived because I couldn't eat a piece of Black Forest cake. I couldn't be a glutton and finish off a pizza at midnight. There was a whole section of the food market that was completely closed off now. All of that was taken away from me. It's not a big thing, but life is demanding enough and this just adds to it.

John's son, a doctor, was a tremendous source of information and advice:

I was fortunate because my son could answer the questions that I had. There was no mystery surrounding diabetes. My son clarified everything. My own doctor didn't have the time to deal with the overwhelming emotional response that diabetes triggered. I remember my son saying that, if I had to pick a disease, diabetes is the healthiest one. He explained that the things I had to do to control diabetes would probably help me take better care of myself than the non-diabetic person in terms of weight control and diet. Looking back I realize how much his comments helped.

From the way John described his reaction to the diagnosis it was apparent that his attitude towards life in general was a great advantage to him. He described how he had watched a friend allow his life to be dominated by illness. John did not want this to happen to him because he enjoyed life too much. With his son's help he realized that he could still live a full life, even though there were adjustments to be made.

Sheila

Sheila was sixty-two when she developed diabetes. It took her a number of years to accept the significance of the diagnosis. She first became aware that something was wrong when she was on holiday, visiting her relatives:

I felt groggy and sick. My relatives said to me, 'You're not very happy. Do you feel well?' I wasn't enjoying my holidays. I was tired all the time. My friends complained that all I wanted to do was drink and sleep. Then I got a bad irritation in the vagina. I didn't know what was causing it.

As soon as Sheila returned home, she followed her relatives' advice and saw her doctor. She discovered that she had diabetes:

I was shocked when the doctor told me I had diabetes. I knew there was something wrong, but it didn't dawn on me that it was diabetes. I really didn't know much about diabetes. I just looked at him and asked him how it could happen. I didn't know what to make of it. I was scared and frightened that I would have to take the needle.

Both of Sheila's brothers had died recently. She speculated about the significance of this upsetting experience for the onset of her diabetes:

My two brothers died at the same time. It was quite an upset. I don't know whether it's true or not that a shock could bring diabetes on. I didn't really know too much about it. No one in our family had diabetes, so I guess it doesn't have to be hereditary. Anyone can get it.

Sheila's doctor told her that she was susceptible to diabetes because of her age and weight. Overweight had been a problem for Sheila. Getting used to the diabetes meal plan was difficult. Sheila's love of food and her reputation as a good cook interfered with the diet. She also had trouble following the diet because she did not understand it:

My doctor sent me to a dietitian, but I couldn't seem to grasp these exchanges. I didn't seem to progress too well. I'd be doing fine and all of a sudden I'd go right off the wagon, not realizing what it was all about.

Sheila was also caring for her elderly father-in-law when she developed diabetes, which made demands on her time and energy. The combination of stress at work, responsibilities at home, a lack of knowledge about the diet, and a love of food all contributed to Sheila's inability to come to terms with diabetes at the time of diagnosis. It was not until her father-in-law died and she retired that Sheila took the time to learn more about diabetes. She found a dietitian who helped her understand the diet and who realized how difficult it was for her to lose weight. This support enabled her to control her weight. Sheila commented on the changes she made as a result:

I never took it seriously when I first had diabetes. I used to think, 'Will it ever go away?' It took me a while to understand what could happen and how important it is. It's something you can't play around with. I got into the habit of eating. I had to keep saying to myself, 'You've got to change.' It takes time to change. Diabetes just stays with you, so you have to learn to live with it.

The diagnosis of diabetes did not have a strong impact on Sheila's behaviour. Her story provides an illustration of how long it can take before a person accepts the need to change behaviour. Other stresses demanded more of Sheila's attention than her health. It was not until these stresses disappeared that she placed a priority on diabetes and began to take better care of herself.

Summary

In most cases people had no cause to suspect that the reason they were feeling unwell was because of diabetes. Frequently the symptoms, especially the excessive fatigue, were attributed to stress and were ignored as long as possible. Once diagnosed, most people reacted with shock and dismay. They wondered why they developed it. Those who had a family history of diabetes suspected it was the cause of their symptoms and were better prepared to face its implications. A determination to get on with living and to take one day at a time helped people begin the adjustment phase. The intensity of the emotional reactions experienced by people was fuelled by their ignorance about the condition. Learning more about diabetes helped to ease the impact as did support from family and friends.

The issues people grappled with initially were the same ones that continued to confront them over the following months and years as they learned to integrate diabetes into their lives. These issues – learning more about the condition, getting on with working and socializing, discovering the value of support, and ultimately gaining control over diabetes are all discussed in more detail in the following chapters.

EXERCISES

You have read how seven people responded to the diagnosis of diabetes. People described their symptoms, their reactions, and their experiences as they adjusted to the condition. Some also discussed what helped them cope in the weeks following diagnosis.

The following exercises are directed towards two different groups. The first set of questions, (A), is meant for people who have had diabetes for longer than six months. The second set of questions, (B), borrows many of the ideas from the first set but is intended for those of you who have been recently diagnosed. All exercises are suitable for either individual or group use.

A / For individuals who have had diabetes longer than six months

1 / *Where have I been: Where do I go?*

Use the opportunity of recalling the period around diagnosis to help you clarify where you currently stand vis-à-vis diabetes. This clarity may a) help you assess whether you wish to make changes or b) simply help you see how far you have come and how much you have learned since your diagnosis.

There are three parts to this exercise. Part (a) will help you recall the circumstances of your diagnosis. Part (b) will help you draw comparisons between how things were then and how they are now. Then in Part (c) you summarize what you have learned and consider changes or actions you might wish to pursue.

a / Your case

Write brief notes in answer to each of these questions:

- What words or phrases would you use to describe your feelings at the time of diagnosis? Try to remember key remarks you made and the things you did when you learned of your condition.
- Once you were diagnosed, what was the turning point in 'getting on with it'?
- What adjustments did you make immediately? Soon after? (Think of diet, exercise, schedule, social life, other activities.)
- How did your family react? Your friends? Was there any person whose reaction was especially important?
- What impact, if any, did your diagnosis have upon work? You could use these answers to write a vignette for yourself like one of those in this chapter.

b / Then and now comparison

Prepare a chart as shown below divided into KEY IDEAS, THEN, and NOW. Use the questions in the chart to fill it out. Write down words or short phrases that catch the reactions and experiences you had then and your reactions and experiences now.

KEY IDEAS	THEN	NOW
Emotions	How did I feel?	How do I feel now?
Fears and fantasies	What was the worst thing that was going to happen to me?	Did it happen? What are your worst fears now?
Family/friends	Who helped? Who didn't? What were their reactions?	Who helps? Who doesn't? What are their reactions now?

Successes/ frustrations	What went well/ badly?	What is going well/badly now?
Actions	What did I do? What could I not do? What did I stop doing? What did I avoid doing?	What can I do? What can't I do? What do I avoid?

c / Summarize your answers by completing these sentences:

- Then I used to believe _____

- But now I know that _____

- I have found out that _____

- I can handle diabetes better now because _____

- Life is better/worse, easier/harder because _____

- I can consider changing _____

2 / My pearls of wisdom

This exercise provides another approach to assessing what you have learned about diabetes since the time of diagnosis. Write a letter to an imaginary person who has recently been diagnosed as having diabetes. Share your experiences around the time of diagnosis. Talk about some of the following things:
- what helped you cope and what got in the way
- what you would recommend she/he avoid doing
- what you suggest she/he do
- what worked for you

- the major things you learned
- the things you found difficult to deal with and how you coped with them
- the things you would do differently
- helpful advice you received from others
- what you wish you had been told at the time
- where you think you are now with diabetes
- where you would like to be in the future

If you know someone who has recently developed diabetes you might consider sharing this with her/him.

B / For individuals who have had diabetes six months or less

1 / Where am I: Where do I want to go?

a / Write brief notes in answer to each of these questions:

- What words or phrases describe how you are feeling about diabetes and its impact on your life?
- What adjustments did you make immediately? Now? (Think of diet, exercise, schedule, social life, other activities.)
- How is your family reacting? Your friends? Is there any person whose reaction is very important to you? Why?
- What impact is diabetes having on your work?

b / How am I doing?

Prepare a chart as shown below divided into KEY IDEAS and WHAT'S HAPPENING. Use the questions in the chart to fill it out. Write down words or share phrases that catch your reactions and experiences.

KEY IDEAS	WHAT'S HAPPENING
Emotions	How do I feel?
Fears and fantasies	What are the worst things that can happen to me?
Family/friends	Who is helping? Who isn't? What would I like from them?
Successes/frustrations	What is going well for me? What is going badly for me?
Actions	What have I done? What have I stopped doing? What can I not do? What do I want to do? What can I do?

c / Summarize your answers by completing these sentences:

- I have found out that _____

- Life is better/worse, easier/harder because _____

- I can't handle diabetes because _____

- I can handle diabetes because _____

- I can consider changing _____

2 / Will things change?

Find someone who has had diabetes for a number of years and ask if you can interview him or her. Think about questions that will help you learn about what is to come. You might wish to use some of the questions from Part A, Exercise 2 (My pearls of wisdom) above.

CHAPTER FOUR

Learning to cope

Introduction

Once the initial shock of diagnosis receded, our participants tried to grasp the implications of diabetes. Almost immediately they received some form of instruction about what diabetes was and what they should be doing to control it. It was then their responsibility to fit the tasks of diabetes management into their regular pattern of living. Despite the teaching, people felt uncertain about their own abilities to cope effectively. As they tried to make changes they often discovered that some things related to diabetes management conflicted with other daily practices and with deep-seated values and beliefs. Many talked about feelings of deprivation and loss. Some people made the recommended changes in their personal lives to accommodate the treatment routine, while others experimented to find approaches that were less disruptive to their established way of life. It was not uncommon for people to experiment with both routes of change in the search for a comfortable compromise. They had to experience these changes before they could judge the impact on their everyday lives.

Our participants were slowly learning about the personal implications of having diabetes in these initial stages of adjustment. These implications could not be learned from health professionals or by reading books. It was something people could really only discover and learn to deal with through their experiences of living with the condition every day.

What does it mean? What do I do?

As we saw in Chapter 3, the diagnosis of diabetes triggered feelings of uncertainty and confusion in the people we interviewed. They were not sure about their next step. The degree of confusion depended partly on the adequacy of the initial teaching. When teaching was limited it was difficult to appreciate the seriousness of the condition or to know what to do. For example, the instructions Sheila received were sparse and did not inspire self-confidence:

In the beginning I really wasn't schooled on what I should do. I knew nothing. The doctor gave me pills and told me to lay off the salt because of my high blood pressure. He sent me to a dietitian. She just threw me this book and said, 'Follow it, the exchanges are there.' I couldn't make head or tail of the book, and it frustrated me more than it did me any good. I went right off the diet.

Jennifer had similar problems:

It never crossed my mind it could be such a serious illness. The doctor gave me the pills and I was okay. It didn't affect me that much. I knew there was some kind of connection between the pills and sugar, but I didn't know how the pills were working. I thought they worked like aspirin. If you have a headache you take an aspirin and it goes away. Diabetes meant nothing to me.

Inadequate teaching was more of a problem for non-insulin-dependent individuals because they were rarely hospitalized or sent immediately to diabetes-education programs. In contrast, those who required insulin were usually diagnosed in hospital. Here they were generally given detailed instructions on how to control diabetes and how to monitor their blood sugar level. A family member frequently was given instructions as well. This was particularly important if the family member was involved in meal preparation. Hospitalization, however, does not guarantee competent instruction. Lynn, for example, received very little information and minimal encouragement while in the hospital:

The diabetes specialist that diagnosed me said that diabetes was a pain in the neck. Then he said I would probably be a lot healthier than a lot of my friends and probably live to be a good age. I was told I had to take insulin once a day. I was given the book that explained the diet and told to be careful not to eat too much and, if I felt like it, I should exercise a little. That was it, finished!

Predictably, Lynn went home discouraged:

When I left hospital I went home and ate a half a box of cookies and thought, 'What am I going to do now? How am I going to follow all that stuff?'

Comprehensive instructions could ease the uncertainty and worry by building confidence about coping on one's own. Gwyn got off to a good start:

I learned what diabetes was all about and how to look after myself. Knowing this allowed me to adjust to having diabetes. The more I learned about it, the more I could cope with it. They say that it's not all that bad – there are bright spots ahead. You can live with it. I was able to look at diabetes more objectively. I think it was a good start.

Yet many people expressed apprehension about applying what they had learned. In the face of day-to-day living our participants quickly realized that they had just begun the real learning:

In the hospital you're in a very sheltered environment. There's no activity, and your food is being looked after. There is a lot of support. Then you come home and you are faced with the realistic part of life. You've got to do your own shopping and your own activities. I walked into the house and I burst into tears. I thought, 'Oh my gosh, look what I've got to live with now. Here I'm faced with looking after myself for the rest of my life.' It was frightening!

The reality of diabetes

In the months following diagnosis the realities of coping with diabetes emerged. The three aspects of diabetes management that were frequently described as difficult to adjust to were the unpredictable swings in blood sugar, the restrictions and regimentation, especially those related to the diet, and the ongoing, long-term nature of the management tasks.

Unpredictability

Regulating the level of blood sugar was frequently a difficult process, and the majority of people we interviewed spoke at length about the limitations and frustrations they encountered. The unpredictability of diabetes was one of their more profound frustrations. This was especially true for those who were insulin-dependent. Following the prescribed treatment did not guarantee normal blood glucose levels. Sometimes, participants developed an insulin reaction or very high blood glucose levels for no apparent reason. Repeatedly, they examined their actions in minute detail. They struggled to find the key to these unpredictable swings in blood sugar. Tim described the process:

I'm always looking at myself asking, 'What am I doing? Am I doing it right? I wonder how long the effect of exercise is supposed to last? How much did I really burn off or how much do I compensate? What do I have to eat?' I don't want to overeat. But then again, I don't want to fall into reactions. I'm trying to find the in-between. It's very tough.

In many cases, through trial and error and consultations with health professionals, participants learned to find the 'in-between.' They learned to estimate the effect of exercise and the impact of stress. But many people had to accept that there were times when their body's response was simply unpredictable. Their best efforts could not change that fact:

Part of the frustration is that, while things go reasonably well, it's not perfect. Doing everything right doesn't guarantee that blood sugars won't go up. I've been unable to constantly keep blood sugars in the normal range. I am doing all that I can – the diet, and exercise, multiple insulin doses, and I don't always get the kind of control I want.

Restrictions and regimentation

Fortunately, for most people these sudden, unexplained changes in their metabolism did not happen frequently enough to seriously hamper their activity. Nonetheless, other

annoyances persist. Two sources of irritation that were discussed at length were the dietary restrictions and the
imposition of a regimented lifestyle.

Everyone who has diabetes faces dietary restrictions. Each
person missed eating certain foods. It was common for people
to say to us, 'If I didn't have diabetes I would eat ...' and complete the sentence with the food or foods they missed the
most.

Food preferences and food habits are closely linked to our
family histories and to cultural norms. When the diabetes diet
conflicts with values we have adopted over time then the necessary changes are difficult. Jennifer's case illustrates this
point:

*My kids were telling me that I must lose weight saying,
'Mother, you're going to kill yourself.' You are actually
killing yourself slowly but it's so hard to diet. I've been
hungry for so many years, living through World War II for
six years and then two years in Russia. You take food for
granted when you're young. We didn't have the food. Four
years in Germany was tremendously difficult. I promised
myself afterward that I'm never going to starve myself
again.*

The North American culture emphasizes the consumption
of food. Fast foods and eating in restaurants have become a
way of life. At the same time food preparation and eating
have become associated with leisure, pleasure, and self-
expression. As many have discovered, dieting under such
circumstances is not easy. Sheila spoke for others when she
said:

*I've always enjoyed my food. I love to eat. Dieting is hard
whether it's for diabetes or losing weight. One of my joys
was enjoying my food. I always liked trying new recipes. I*

*miss that part of it as well as not being able to eat
everything that you want.*

Another complaint was a loss of spontaneity and pleasure.
Food became a form of treatment, like medicine. It lost its
more enjoyable features:

*Diet and food are the most repressive parts of diabetes.
You eat what you need, when you need it, and in correct
amounts. You have to eat it, even if you don't want it. It's
completely opposite to normal eating. You eat according to
plan, not hunger or desire.*

*Hunger, appetite, and cravings have absolutely nothing to
do with the diabetic way of eating. That is depressing,
because hunger and appetite are normal functions of the
human body. You get hungry for something and you satisfy yourself. Now I feel more like a machine. It's like
input and output. I feel like the basic function of my body
has been taken away from me.*

In addition to the restrictions, there was the challenge of
adhering to a routine regimen. This aspect was frequently
more frustrating than coping with a restricted diet. Balancing
diet and insulin by consuming meals and snacks at regular
times made many people feel as if their lives were pro-
grammed:

*You must regulate your life with precision; breakfast at
seven, snack at ten-thirty, lunch at twelve, dinner at seven
and evening snack at ten-thirty. You constantly have to
test your blood. Those things become uppermost and then
it's difficult to live in the cracks.*

*Diabetes really rules my life. My whole life has become
very structured and scheduled. It interferes with the life I*

want to live, but it's a matter of trying to live a reasonable life. I have time frames and I'm allowed to do things within certain time frames. Because of the type of diabetes I have, being a structured person is important to good management. Other diabetics might not have to be so pristine in their existence.

Those who desired spontaneity complained that living by a routine was boring. They missed the freedom to act on impulse; to enjoy, for example, the simple pleasure of a snack consumed because of a whim instead of necessity.

The need for a routine meant that almost all activities required advance planning; there was no room for foul-ups or even a carefree attitude. Gary cited a typical example:

I have to follow a fairly rigid diet of times and amounts. That's limiting. I can't go sailing for a day, forget to take lunch, and come back and have a couple of beers and a sandwich like I used to.

No escape

When Gary said, 'I can't forget,' he identified a key feature of diabetes. Diabetes is an unavoidable part of life:

One of the hindrances of living with diabetes is the endless living with it, in itself. You go on and on! It's hard to escape – you really don't ever have a vacation.

The ongoing demands of diabetes meant that the management tasks were viewed as 'work' and there were times when it was wearisome. Furthermore, the need to continuously assess and monitor their own situation was tiring:

I always have to be aware, I always have to think. It really tires you out mentally. Sometimes it gets quite exhausting.

Despite the mental fatigue, the irritations with routines, the difficulties of following a diet, and the uncertainties surrounding diabetes control, people learned to cope. They faced life one day at a time and by trial and error learned to master diabetes.

The learning process

Much of the initial learning about how to cope came through experience. The process is akin to learning to swim by leaping into the water. This is one of the ways participants developed techniques to help minimize the impact of diabetes. In addition, many people had to experiment with guidelines to see how far they could push the limits of diabetes control. Ultimately, they had to learn to exercise their own judgment to find the path that enabled them to manage the condition and still live a life that was personally satisfying.

Trial and error

I had a lot of questions that people around me had answers to, but I needed to answer them myself. I had to have the experience to be able to say to myself, 'Okay, now I know what I can do and what I can't do.'

In the statement above, Gwyn summarizes what others also discovered about learning to cope – that is, experience is the best teacher. The lessons were sometimes learned the hard way, yet most believed first hand experience was the best way to learn how to be personally responsible.

Sometimes the learning could be quite straightforward, as in Nancy's case, when she learned the importance of being prepared for insulin reactions:

I had my first insulin reaction when we were on a vacation. We had gone to an exercise program that morning.

When we got back to the hotel room, my husband suggested we go for a walk because we had an hour before lunch. I always carry candy in my purse but I didn't think I was going to need it because we were only going for a short walk. I didn't realize that I had just done a bit too much. When you do extra activity, you are supposed to compensate with extra food. I hardly made it back from the walk. It was very frightening. After that I wouldn't go anywhere unless I carried something with me.

More often, the learning represents an accumulation of experiences. Over a period of time people figure out ways to make difficult changes. For example, changing eating patterns means learning new ways to deal with food. In the following examples Sheila and Michael both illustrate how with time, and by trial and error they learned to control their eating:

I need self-control with food. If I get upset I'll find that I'll start picking at food, but I'm learning to control it, to do something else. I'll go and watch the news on TV and get lost in that and forget all about what upset me, or I'll pick up a book and start reading. I don't keep anything sweet in the house that I think is going to tempt me. You get depressed and say, 'I'm going to have some of that.' I got to the stage that, when people gave me chocolates, I gave them to somebody else as soon as their backs were turned. The whole box would go. I just get them out of the house because, if I opened them and took one, then I'm at them all the time.

It took a month to get used to the diet. You do little things like, if you're going to have a snack, you bring out the knife and fork, put a plate out, bring everything out, and set the table. You make it trouble to do it. After a while you psychologically adjust yourself to say, 'Why bother,

*it's too much trouble.' And then you don't have anything.
Or if I felt hungry, I'd go out in the garden and do some
weeding just to keep busy. As long as I keep active I can
stay away from food. There's a health club where I work
and I've discovered that if I go there hungry and exercise, I
come out not being hungry anymore. So I got in the habit
of doing that as well, a few times in the week.*

Many people described learning to plan. It became necessary to anticipate and plan for daily events just to ensure
some flexibility. Much of the planning centred around food.
Food had to be available when needed. Some carried additional insulin so they could respond to unexpected circumstances. Planning ahead became a skill. Some people
were 'natural' planners, but others had to learn the process.
Gwyn, for example, said, 'Planning goes very much against
my nature because I am a free and easy type.' She soon discovered that to indulge her needs for flexibility and spontaneity she had no choice but to overcome her resistance to
planning. Eventually it became second nature:

*I have an automatic checklist. I check off all the stuff I
have to do. For example, I consider when meetings are and
what to have for lunch. It is something I didn't do
consciously before.*

Assessing the limits

Assessing the limits of diabetes control was another important part of learning to cope. Some people found this was an
easy task. They simply convinced themselves that they must
accept the imposed limits. Tim captured this philosophy:

*I do get bored with the diet and eating at certain times, but
there is no other way. So when you come to your limit, as*

long as you know there is no other way, it's not so bad. If I knew there were other choices, then it would really bother me, but I know there are none. I've got to put up with this. I either learn to accept it, or it's going to be frustrating. There is no other way. This is what they call the normal way of life for diabetics.

Others chose to test the limits. Some, like Gary, pushed the limits and discovered the consequences were not to their liking:

I was challenging the disease, saying 'What can you do to me if I don't do this?' I found out quickly. I had a few severe reactions. I thought it was foolish that I let this happen. I could have taken corrective, preventive measures. If I had been eating properly, it wouldn't have happened. So I promised myself that it was not going to happen again. I learned that I couldn't carry on with that sort of thing. I had to pay more attention to the diet and eat properly, or at least at regular times.

Still others discovered that life was more satisfying if they bent the rules a bit. Gwyn was determined to be flexible in order to keep a balanced perspective:

I was becoming a crank, thinking, 'I've got to go and do this and I can't stay and do that.' I thought, 'I can't go on living this way,' so I made adjustments so that the diet fit the way I was used to living. There is flexibility in the diet. Each person adapts it to his own system within reason of what has been set out. If you build in such a strict routine, then the longer you do that the more you feel really confined to it. Then you get out of being able to be the least bit flexible. I felt that might happen and I didn't want it to happen.

Some used the term 'cheating' to describe the things they did to stretch the limits. Cheating has a negative connotation as it implies breaking the rules. Viewed more positively, cheating is a way of learning through experimentation. These people were learning to take responsibility, to find the balance that seemed right for them. They tried out certain things and observed the consequences. Then they decided whether or not their actions were too risky. In describing what she learned during her first year with diabetes Elizabeth illustrates this process:

I have gotten the confidence to make up my own mind about things from a combination of experiencing living as a diabetic for a year, getting all the facts and information that I have, and using my own judgment. For example, my husband and I went to Florida. Like an idiot I walked along the beach with my sandals on because I didn't want to cut my foot. Towards the end of the week I took off my sandals. I thought, 'This is ridiculous. The nurses will really yell at me but too bad. It's my life.' I knew what I might be in for and knew that I had to be careful and really watch out for sharp pieces. If I did get a cut I'd wash it out right away. Nothing happened.

You get to the point where you're going to make yourself crazy. My body would be healthy but my mind wouldn't be. I didn't think there was that much risk and I was willing to take it, whereas before I would think, 'I was told I shouldn't do that so I better not do it.'

I'm easing up on things and learning to live with diabetes. I'm not striving for absolute perfection anymore. I'm relaxing with it. The year has taught me a lot. If there is something I absolutely know nothing about, I know I can call the dietitian or I can ask the doctor. If there's something I'm absolutely in doubt about, I wouldn't do it until I have the information I need, but I haven't come across that yet.

Elizabeth's most significant learning was how to use her own judgment when faced with the choices encountered in daily living. She learned that she must assess risks for herself and reach her own decisions if she wished to lead a satisfying life. She learned to temper advice from health professionals by using common sense. Finally, Elizabeth learned to relax. She recognized that with time, the combination of information from others, personal experience, and the use of judgment would lead to successful coping.

Self-monitoring

Until recently is was difficult to know how certain factors affected diabetes control. However, the introduction of home blood glucose monitoring devices has changed that situation. These devices can provide immediate and reliable feedback on blood glucose levels. One participant commented that when the feedback was 'bad' there was motivation to 'get into line.'

Effects of normal living (fatigue, nervousness, anxiety, and bodily responses to heat and humidity) are often similar to the symptoms of hyper- and hypoglycemia. Blood glucose monitoring devices enabled participants to make distinctions among the symptoms:

If I get up and I feel off and I wonder if this is the diabetes or if it's a typical off-day, then I immediately test before I draw any conclusions.

Nobody's body is the same two days in a row. That's what makes blood glucose monitoring superior to any other way of managing diabetes. Anything can elevate my blood sugar – something physical, premenstrual, postmenstrual, a fight with my kids or my husband, stress. With blood glucose monitoring I can tell if my blood sugar is in a certain range, and then I take 'X' amount of insulin.

Individuals enthusiastically described the increased security and confidence they felt by using this device. The following excerpt captures the sentiments of most:

Blood glucose monitoring gives me more control over my life. With it I'm living a more normal life in the sense that, if I have any doubts about my diabetes, I can go to the machine and two minutes later I'll know exactly what it is.

Summary

We have seen how our participants learned to cope with diabetes on a daily basis. After recovering from the initial shock of diagnosis they began to assess the impact on their lives. The word 'frustration' cropped up frequently in our conversations. Diabetes was unpredictable. Good behaviour did not guarantee good blood sugar control. There was the loss of favourite foods and the difficulties of following a diet in a culture obsessed with food. The regimen interfered with spontaneity, and worst of all, there was no escape. Our participants persevered and learned to cope with many of these constraints. A major part of this learning involved accepting responsibility for managing the condition. This could happen only if they made their own decisions. Decision-making requires judgment and judgment develops with experience. To develop sound judgment many of our participants tested the limits of diabetes control. They weighed professional advice, their own needs, and the consequences of their actions and made judgments about how to live. They developed a greater sense of security and confidence in their ability to manage diabetes and lead a full life.

EXERCISES

This chapter deals with two facets of learning, first, *what* people learned about diabetes and, second, *how* they learned these things. We have selected the exercises that follow because they will help you with both the 'what' and the 'how.' We begin with the 'how.'

A / Helping you learn

Before you begin you may find it helpful to reread Chapter 1 to remind yourself of the different ways we can learn. Then try the exercises that follow. They have been chosen to help you be creative in your approaches to learning. Remember, it is not necessary to complete all of the exercises at one sitting. Read through all the exercises, select one to do now, and save the others until later. Allow yourself time between exercises to think about them. You may find you will want to change or expand some of your answers.

1 / Barriers to learning

There are many factors that hinder learning: poor light, distractions, feelings of anger or resentment, the presence of other people, a lack of resources. Rule a page into two columns entitled HELPS and HINDRANCES. List all the factors that help you and then list all the factors that hinder you from learning about diabetes. Be imaginative. Does it help if you are happy? Ask others for their advice about your lists. (Don't forget to place 'asking others' on your list.)

When you have written your lists, read them over. You may find ways to improve your learning immediately. Develop a learning plan that takes full advantage of the HELPS and minimizes the HINDRANCES. Do you need to do something to get rid of the HINDRANCES? If so – do it!

2 / Finding your own answers: The funnel and the diamond

In his book *The Three Boxes of Life*, Richard Bolles describes how to discover your own answers through a kind of informed research process. The techniques suggested here are based on his approach.

One method involves starting with a broad picture or overview and then narrowing the topic until you can ask and find answers to specific questions. This approach resembles an inverted triangle or a funnel.

A second method is the reverse of the first. It begins with a narrowly defined question or idea. Then you spread the search to develop your own broad picture. (This process resembles a triangle.) Then if you like you can use the first method to again narrow the search like a funnel. These two phases resemble a diamond.

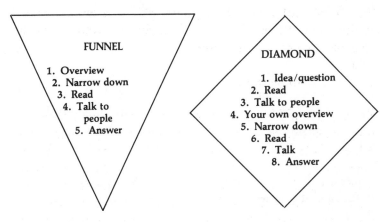

FUNNEL
1. Overview
2. Narrow down
3. Read
4. Talk to people
5. Answer

DIAMOND
1. Idea/question
2. Read
3. Talk to people
4. Your own overview
5. Narrow down
6. Read
7. Talk
8. Answer

Here are some hints for each of the steps of the funnel and of the diamond.

Overview

The best way to get an overview might be an educational program for beginners. You get the big picture, even if it seems vague and general. Sometimes the overview will be in a book. Sometimes you may not find an overview until part way through your search.

Narrowing down

It often helps to spell out what you *don't* want to know. You contract or narrow down the subject matter. You might even do this when you read this book. 'Help and support' is not what you are looking for? Don't read that chapter. Use indexes and tables of contents; look for specifics.

Read

Use the library; use you local diabetes association; ask your doctor for pamphlets. Check the dates to see if materials are current, dated, or out of date. Look for books on similar topics, e.g. other chronic illnesses, that might have relevance to your situation.

Talk to people

Find experts (your doctor, nurses, others with diabetes, dietitians, and so on). Use them to check for accuracy and to try out new ideas and questions. Whenever you talk to someone, ask them for names of other people who could help you.

These are the four essential steps. You can start anywhere but you may find it helpful to set out to learn in a systematic manner.

3 / Sign a contract with yourself

Many people learn better with clear simple goals (was that on your list of helps in the first exercise?). In order to help your learning, write out a brief contract. State the following:

a / What I will learn (the goal – keep it simple).

b / When I will learn it (set a date).

c / How I will know I have learned (specify indicators of achievement).

d / My reward (why not?).

e / How I will do it (strategy, tools, helpers).

f / Signature (commit yourself).

Put your contract in a safe place and take it out when the time is up. Some people like to put the contract in a letter and give it to a friend to mail back on the deadline date. It may help you to have a witness sign the contract, too.

This method is also helpful if you are working with one other person or a group. Write out a contract with each other and assign the rewards to each other for successful completion.

4 / Problem-solving and planning

The Force Field Analysis technique was devised to help people change certain behaviours. It was first used to help people learn to use cheap cuts of meat during World War II. It can work for you as well. It is based on the idea that situations are never really fixed or static. They can be changed. There are various factors that influence a situation and to change the situation, these must be changed. The factors influencing a situation can be thought of as *driving forces* and *restraining forces*. They both exert pressure on your situation and determine the 'status quo' (the situation as it now exists). If you want to change the status quo you need to make a change in the balance created by these forces. Often the easiest way to make changes is to minimize or remove some of the restraining forces. Then the positive pressure of the driving forces will shift you from the status quo (A) to a new, more desirable situation (B).

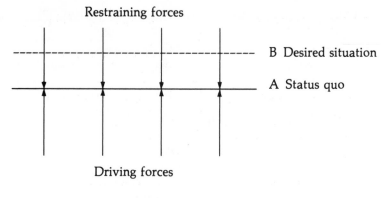

THE FORCE FIELD

Use the following steps to try out this technique.

a / Describe the present situation. A – (I can't manage my diet and play hockey).

b / Describe the desired situation. B – (I will manage my diet and play hockey).

c / Make a chart like the one on page 63 and fill in all the factors or forces that are affecting the present situation. Identify those positive forces that could create change – the driving forces. Identify those that prevent change – the restraining forces. Try to avoid listing statements that are the equivalents of one another (driving = need four meals, restraining = don't get four meals).

d / Look at the restraining forces. How can one or more of them be removed?

e / A good way to remove or reduce restraining forces is to 'brainstorm' all the ideas you can think of about how to get rid of them. To brainstorm you make a list of twenty to thirty ideas for each restraining force you picked. In brainstorming you list every thought you get, even the silly ones – especially the silly ones! Then go back over the list and pick out the good ideas you can use to build a plan to reduce this force. Repeat this exercise for each restraining force. Star the most promising ideas.

DRIVING FORCES	(A)	RESTRAINING FORCES
– My desire to play		– Games are at different hours
– Help from a dietitian		– Extended exertion brings quick drops in sugar
– My experience at hockey games		
– Knowing when I'm getting low sugar		– I feel embarrassed having reactions
– My girlfriend likes hockey		– My coach doesn't know I have diabetes
– Orange juice helps		– I haven't planned my meals before

f / Once you have identified the ideas to work on to remove the restraining forces, make a list of actions you must take to ensure getting rid of them. Write a contract (as in Exercise 3) and get on with it. Good luck!

B / **Coping with the difficulties**

Much of the learning that we read about in this chapter centred around learning what diabetes meant to people in day-to-day living. The primary concerns were related to the restrictions that diabetes imposed and the stuggle to minimize these. The two exercises that follow are designed to help you examine the personal significance of these restrictions and to identify ways to counterbalance them.

1 / Restrictions and how to handle them

We all have restrictions placed on us for one reason or another. Focus on those you have because of diabetes. Here

are seven categories you may wish to use. Write them down the side of a piece of paper. List three or four restrictions you have next to each one of them.
- Daily routine
- Diet and eating habits
- My family
- Other relationships
- Work
- Play
- The way I'm treated
- Not knowing

After you have made your list, divide your restrictions into three other categories.

a / I am controlling ...
b / I can learn to control ...
c / I can't control ...

You now have a good learning agenda. As you learn to control restrictions, you can move them from list (b) to list (a). You also have a learning agenda in list (c). Ask yourself how you can learn to live with things you can't control. Anticipate how you will react. Can you identify ways you can either control or minimize your reactions?

2 / Option B's

Planning is an important aspect of coping effectively with diabetes. It helps lessen the impact of the restrictions. Here is a planning exercise, based on one described by Bolles, that will help you identify options to ease the burdens of diabetes.

In many situations, you plan to do things in a certain way or at a certain time, but things don't work out. If your first plan (Choice A) doesn't work, or is unsatisfactory to you, it might help to have an alternative plan ready. We suggest that you develop an Option B. Try out this approach to see if Option B's will work for you.

At the end of each day for one week, write down the decisions you faced that were related in some way to diabetes and the choices you made. For example, recall how you handled your diet at a dinner party, an invitation for a late lunch, an unexpected deadline at work, or an invitiation to play squash. List all the decisions or choices you made in Column A. Then in Column B, try to invent another set of choices you could have used if Choice A had failed or if you simply would have preferred a different alternative.

CHOICE A   OPTION B
I decided to ...   I could have ...

At the end of the week, decide if anticipating and planning Option B's would help you to cope better.

CHAPTER FIVE

The broader impact of diabetes

Introduction

The impact of diabetes went well beyond the personal frustrations that were described in Chapter 4. Our participants talked a lot about how diabetes affected relationships within the family unit, their social activities and interactions, and their work lives.

There were many instances where diabetes had little or no effect on families. Family members accepted the presence of diabetes and were negatively affected only if the condition was out of control. On the other hand, families already under stress often did not respond well when one member developed diabetes. Under these circumstances the difficulties of coping effectively were compounded by the already complex family situation. A small minority of people discussed the influence of diabetes on sexual function and these are presented at the end of this section.

Social interactions outside the immediate family sometimes posed problems because some people were reluctant to admit that they had diabetes. They worried about being stereotyped in a negative way. Likewise, diabetes could be a significant factor in the workplace. People had to decide whether to discuss diabetes with their colleagues when applying for jobs, or when they were hired. Job discrimination because of diabetes remains a problem. One participant's experience of this will be presented, as will the range of ways in which people learned to control diabetes in the work setting.

Diabetes in the family

Most people did not believe that diabetes had a marked impact on the quality of their family life. They described the response of family members as 'matter-of-fact' and with one exception saw no reason why diabetes would be considered a hindering factor in the day-to-day life of the family. The one exception that some participants discussed was the 'low moods' that accompanied poor control or insulin reactions. Roger's diabetes had been out of control for a number of years and he recalled the impact of his behaviour on his family during that time:

All families of diabetics take a beating to some extent. During my low periods, because of lack of energy and stressful situations, I became almost unbearable. All my attitudes were negative. I could bearly contain myself during the business day and I would come home without any energy at night.

Roger and others recognized that their families exercised restraint under such circumstances. Family members realized that the irritability they observed was related to diabetes and made allowances.

Diabetes posed more problems for families who were under stress before one member developed the condition. When this was the case, coping with diabetes was much more difficult. Pat's situation is a good example. Diabetes was diagnosed when she was thirteen. She was twenty-four when she was interviewed and she was still struggling to cope effectively. Pat summed up the situation during her teenage years:

It sure makes a difference if your parents care. You need a good team behind you. I had no support in the house and I definitely didn't have it out of the house.

Pat believed that her parents were uninterested in her general welfare and indifferent to her diabetes. Her father refused to give her money to buy insulin. Her mother did not help her with her diet. At fifteen she was anorexic. She was frequently hospitalized for poor control. Her doctor encouraged her to leave home, which she eventually did. She frequently relied on social assistance benefits for help. In recent years she has alternated between welfare and working. With the help of her physicians she is beginning to come to terms with diabetes. She has been seeing a psychiatrist for seven years and in the last year has found it very helpful. The physicians she sees at the hospital clinic have all expressed interest, concern, and encouragement. At the present time they are her primary source of support. The following quote speaks well for the health care system, but is a sad commentary on her family:

My experiences at the hospital have shown me that there are people who do care. If your family doesn't care there are people that care. I don't just have to depend on my family anymore. They weren't there for me in the beginning, and they're not there for me now.

Pat's story was the most dramatic example of how a complex family situation complicates coping with diabetes. There were other examples as well. In Catherine's situation her family life was not particularly troubled. Nonetheless, the values expressed in the family had a marked influence on Catherine's response to diabetes. She has had a difficult time accepting diabetes, particularly because she sought perfect control and could not attain it. After twenty-four years she still resents the condition and has not resolved her feelings of anger. In reviewing her upbringing she now sees the impact of what she labels 'Calvinist values.' She was discouraged from express- ing her feelings about the condition; when she did they were discounted. Self-pity was frowned upon. Catherine was expected to maintain control; expressions of approval were contingent on her success. Failure was viewed as a personal shortcoming and meant a fall from grace. Twenty-four years later Catherine is struggling to moderate the influence of the values she grew up with so she can take a more relaxed approach to diabetes.

Both of these examples show the significance of the family in cases of juvenile-onset diabetes. Even when people develop diabetes as adults, coping is complicated by family stress. Carol's situation is similar to Pat's. The condition is not the cause of family difficulties. Instead it is the family problems that make coping more difficult. Diabetes provides one more arena in which family tensions can be played out. Carol cited a typical example:

It's not a happy relationship around here for financial rea- sons. My husband does the shopping. It's what he needs, not what I need. My needs and wants don't matter. Lots of times I don't have the things in the house to eat that I should be eating. I have to play it by ear and I do eat things I shouldn't be eating, simply for the fact there isn't anything else here that suits my diet.

In Susan's case diabetes was simply more difficult to con- trol because of the tension between her and her husband, much of which was generated by problems with their children:

The stress is my family. I've discovered something I don't like the implications of. My husband was away for a trip this summer and my sugar was down while he was away.

We're fine on our own; it's when the kids are around or having problems that we have trouble.

One facet of diabetes that is rarely discussed is the impact of diabetes on sexual function. Very few of our participants discussed the relationship between diabetes and sexual function. Of the few who did, most knew that diabetes could occasionally lead to impotence in men. Concern was expressed that health professionals were reluctant to broach the issue. We are including a brief section on this topic with the hope that it might encourage more open discussion.

We talked to only one person who described difficulties with impotence. He said:

Sex and potency is a very embarrassing subject. It is very personal. Diabetes is tied in with a lessened potency. It is a bit applicable to me; not a lot, thank goodness. That adjustment can be demoralizing for a male. It is something men don't talk about openly. It's come out in talking to some friends with diabetes. One friend was not aware that many others have the same problem. He thought it was him. He was more concerned about impotency than diabetes. I reassured him that it was not abnormal. I was searching for the right words to make him a man again in his own mind. A male feels that if he's impotent you've taken his manhood.

He also stressed the need for a more open discussion of the problem:

It's better knowing than not knowing. Otherwise you think you are dealing with two burdens, impotency and diabetes. It helps to know the two are the same. You make adjustments but with resignation. It's like they have chopped away something else again. It's a loss.

The other men who spoke of impotence knew that decreased sexual function could be attributed to the lethargy and fatigue associated with both very high and very low blood glucose levels. This fact reinforced for them the need to keep diabetes under control.

While the complications of diabetes can lead to impotence in men, its influence in women is less certain. The few women who commented on sexuality and diabetes said that diabetes had not influenced their sexual function or pleasure. Catherine, however, like the men described above, found it another motivator for maintaining good control:

I've only seen one study having to do with women, which was many, many years ago. The literature relates to male impotence, but a woman's difficulty in achieving orgasm might be related to blood sugar control – like male impotence. To maintain the pleasure of a good sex life is a very good personal reason for keeping good control.

It is encouraging to see that, for the most part, the people we interviewed encountered few difficulties integrating diabetes with their family lives. Under such circumstances, the family provides a solid base allowing people to shift their attention to their social and work milieus.

Diabetes in the social world

The key issue arising from social interactions was the fear of being labelled 'different.' People disliked being singled out and feared being stereotyped. Most of the people we spoke to wanted to be treated just like everybody else. They did not want any extra attention. On the other hand, coping with diabetes required special effort and self-discipline and they appreciated people who acknowledged their perseverance.

People spoke at length about the differences between their

own activities and behaviours and those of people who did not have diabetes. What others did was 'normal.' What they had to do was 'abnormal.' Still, everybody was quite clear that although their behaviour might be abnormal, 'inside' they were as normal as anybody else:

I don't consider myself different from other people. I suppose I'm somewhat different because of diabetes but I consider myself normal.

I like to think that I am normal except there are some things I have to do to be normal. In somebody else's eyes that's not normal.

Many people suspected that this distinction was not necessarily clear to the general public. They feared being labelled 'handicapped,' 'limited,' or 'damaged.' Some people, in fact, had experiences that fuelled their concern. For example, Dana distinctly remembered that her friends were not allowed to play with her after she developed diabetes:

When I was young, in the late fifties, I remember that mothers would not let me play with their children. They were afraid that diabetes was contagious. The ignorance was unbelievable. If the girl from across the street was playing with my sisters she would have to leave when I came out to play. When I told my mother she said that they didn't understand that diabetes was not contagious. I didn't think there was anything wrong with me, but they thought there was. It took six months for them to get over that. Because of the trauma of these kids not playing with me I think I fought to be supernormal.

Lydia also described two incidents that implied the view that people with diabetes are blemished:

I was standing up in the bus and the girl beside me examined my medic-alert bracelet and then released it as if I had the plague. I thought it was her problem if she thought of me as a leper because I had diabetes. I still think there is a stigma attached to having diabetes. I have a friend who works for an insurance company. She thinks of diabetes in a negative way because, unfortunately, the cases of diabetes that come across her desk involve really bad complications. She was really surprised when she found out that I had it and was able to do what I did.

Some people were annoyed whenever they encountered a public reminder of their condition. They believed this unwanted attention emphasized surface differences between themselves and others and gave them unwanted visibility. Such situations often arose from an inadvertent remark or gesture. For example, Tim resented it when people commented on his snacking pattern:

I feel really self-conscious about it. It bothers me. People don't know that I eat because I have to, not because I want to. I think that I have to explain it to them. I'm supposed to try to live a normal life. I don't consider it normal when I have to explain to somebody why I'm having a snack. It turns me off. I want to sneak the stuff just so I don't have to give them a big explanation.

Elizabeth was disconcerted when an acquaintance forgot she had diabetes and offered her cake, then remembered and apologized:

It's embarrassing. I just said, 'It's okay,' and nothing more was said about it. I guess you get used to it, but it's like being pointed out.

Eventually most people we spoke to accepted that at times they had to be different and stopped worrying about what others thought of them. Although they might not explicitly state they had diabetes they felt comfortable expressing their needs and doing what was necessary to maintain control. For those who still find such an approach difficult Craig offered this hope:

When you get older, it is easier to march to your own drummer. When you're younger, at least for the majority of us, it's much more difficult to be different.

The 'Catch 22'

Although some people were quite clear about not wishing to be singled out others had mixed feelings. They wanted both to be treated 'normally' and to be treated 'specially.' Craig spoke of this contradiction:

I don't want people to make a fuss about me, but then sometimes I'm resentful because they don't make a fuss about me. It's a real screwy deal. First one side and now the other. But the bulk of the time I want to be treated like everybody else.

Sarah elaborated:

Diabetes is part of me as a person and it's something people need to deal with if they're interested in me as a person. On the other hand, if people over-deal with the diabetes part of me I get put in a terrible position. It's embarrassing when someone prepares a whole separate meal for me. I need acknowledgment of it but that kind of attention is embarrassing.

It can be a fine line between lavishing unwelcome attention and failing to notice something that holds special meaning.

In an earlier quote Tim complained about unwanted attention, but at the same time he sought acknowledgment of the hardships he bore:

When nobody asks me how I'm doing, I start to wonder if people think that diabetes is nothing, absolutely nothing! I get the impression that people think that all I have to do is take my needle every day. They seem to think it's so simple. It's almost like insulin is the cure. Boy, if they only knew! They're just not aware of how it really is. They don't realize what I've got to go through every single day.

Telling others

Given many people's sensitivity to the stigma associated with diabetes, it is not surprising that many were reluctant to acknowledge that they had it. Some people were quite open about it, but most avoided telling others and were very selective about whom they told. The rule of thumb appeared to be that you did not broadcast it. Family and close friends were told; others might be told if they asked specific questions.

There was a common belief that diabetes was a very personal aspect of one's life, which would not be revealed to 'just anyone.' It took courage to overcome a fear of making a spectacle of oneself or to contend with a response that was upsetting. With time, however, some people overcame their reluctance to tell others. Sometimes it simply felt better to explain the reasons behind behaviours that were different. Others, like Ellen, thought it was important to stand up and be counted:

I feel it is very important that diabetics stand up for themselves to promote knowledge of diabetes generally and facilities for diabetics. There are so many thousands of us and if more people are knowledgeable and more aware of diabetes if makes it easier for us. Then we won't have to duck the issue or fight ignorance.

Ultimately, it is easier for people to take a public stand on diabetes when they themselves have come to terms with the condition. Lydia and Elizabeth both expressed this point of view:

I have found that I have come to an inner peace about having diabetes. This helps me. If I have to tell people about having diabetes, I don't feel this stigma about it and worry that they are going to hate me for it. My feeling now is that anyone who believes that everybody has to be perfect is wrong.

I find it easier to lay it on the line. I feel more comfortable with it that way. I used to not tell others because I didn't want to be pitied. Now I don't feel afraid of being pitied because I don't feel I pity myself anymore.

At the same time that people were learning to cope with new aspects of their social lives they also had to learn to manage diabetes in the workplace.

Diabetes and work

Difficulties faced in the work world mirrored those of the social setting. Individuals had to decide whether to declare that they had diabetes and if so to determine the best timing. They were concerned about the stigma and believed that it could result in discrimination, both in hiring and in on-the-job practices. On the other hand, it was apparent that the diabetes-related difficulties that emerged at work could, for the most part, be handled effectively by individuals. This was particularly true when the employer displayed flexibility and support.

Discussing diabetes

Because people were concerned about a prospective employer's response to diabetes they questioned if they should talk about it during a job interview. Sometimes they wondered if the fact they had mentioned diabetes was the reason they did not get the job. This concern was heightened during periods when the market was tight and jobs were hard to find. The majority were hesitant to mention diabetes. They believed that under most circumstances, it was not important for the employer to know. Once on the job, it was again necessary to decide whether to raise it. People expressed a range of views about this issue. If an individual developed diabetes while working it was more likely that colleagues would be informed about it. This was true for Tim, who was off work for a considerable time when he developed diabetes:

When I went back to work I explained to the boss that I had diabetes but said it was not going to affect anything I do. I told him that I was going to still be able to perform well for him. My boss said, 'No problem,' and we just carried on. The people in my office were pretty good. I informed them so that if anything happened they would know what to do. I had a bad reaction one morning and that was it – the only time in seven or eight years. The other people who don't work in my office probably don't even know that I have diabetes.

Ian developed diabetes late in his career. He worked as a foreman in a plant. A number of his fellow workers had other health problems, so when he developed diabetes he did not hesitate to tell his boss:

Somebody should definitely know, somebody whom you work with or who is close to you, so that they know what is happening. My boss knows. There was no problem. He wasn't shocked. There is a medical centre at the plant. The nurse knows. You can't fool the company. When people bring in their prescriptions, the nurse knows exactly what those prescriptions are.

Some, like Gwyn, found it more difficult to discuss diabetes because the work related implications were unclear:

It was really hard having to go to work and say to somebody, 'Guess what I found out on Friday!' It was particularly difficult to go to my boss and tell him that I may have to be off work for a while, because I didn't know how much I was going to be able to do. I wondered whether I was going to have to give up my job.

Others chose not to speak about diabetes unless an opportunity arose naturally. Gary said:

When I got the job last year, I did not go around and say, 'I'm a diabetic. If I act a little weird sometimes that's why.' Sometimes just in the course of a conversation an opportunity would arise for me to mention it. Not that I wanted to draw undue attention to it but just so that they would know. The opportunity to tell my boss arose when I had to say I couldn't make it to a meeting he had called unexpectedly because I had a doctor's appointment. I said that it wasn't just a normal doctor's appointment. I had to have a blood sugar test because I'm a diabetic. He asked if I had any problems with it and we had a conversation about it. It was nothing serious.

Then there were people like Dana, who never did reveal that she had diabetes:

If they had known about diabetes at work, I would have had to prove myself even more. At the company where I

*worked there were few females in the higher echelon. I had
to work much harder as a female management person than
a male. If they had known about the condition, it would
have been more difficult to prove myself. They could have
used that as a reason for expecting me to fail or do a lousy
job. I never had any problem with diabetes during the time
I worked. I covered it up a lot. I think I overcompensated
because of not wanting anyone to know. It can be a constantly stressful situation. It is a struggle to remain as normal as possible. Out in the work force, who cares what's
wrong with you as long as you do the job! It shouldn't
matter.*

Discrimination

The fear of discrimination on the job was of concern to a
small number of people. Only two individuals talked about
experiencing overt discrimination at work. Discrimination is
difficult to prove legally. It has a profound and traumatic
effect on its victims. For this reason we are presenting Roger's
story of job discrimination.

Roger was a senior salesperson for an international corporation. He described the business environment in which he
worked as follows:

*In corporate situations in this country senior executives are
heavily involved with alcohol and poor dietary habits.
They eat on the run. Every corporate lunch becomes a
drinking session for two or three hours. This was especially
true for the people in my profession. They have a reputation for heavy drinking and wild living. Unless you are a
member of this fraternity, you are not one of the boys.*

Even after he developed diabetes, Roger continued to be
'one of the boys.' But after years of feeling unwell, he decided
he had to make changes in his lifestyle in order to combat dia-

betes. The changes he made had a significant impact on his business life and were not well received by his colleagues:

I decided to make health my number one priority and started to watch my diet more closely and make sure I followed a routine. This contravened the typical lifestyle of my profession. My colleagues subtly disapproved. For example, when reading the menu at lunch, others would make comments that their specialist in diet, meaning me, might not approve of it.

For the first two or three years I would laugh it off, but it became a very overbearing situation. The disapproval from the senior executives became more direct. They said, 'We really can't bring you to this meeting because we feel your attitude is such that it will disturb the negotiation and the client might be put off.' It reached the point where I was no longer allowed to go to any general sales meetings or any meeting where senior management were present. I was told that they were totally embarrassed by my conduct. They seemed to feel that I'd become a prude because I could no longer relax and drink at the end of meetings. This was all part of their concept of being a successful salesperson. Yet I sold multi-million dollar projects with twenty-five to thirty people in a meeting, and I can think of many occasions where I suggested we adjourn the meeting at noon hour in order to have lunch and the general comment was, 'What an excellent idea, I wish our people would do this.'

I could never understand the difference between the outside world and the environment I was dealing with except that the outside world was made up of strangers and there was a natural courtesy between people. This wasn't the case within the corporation of which I was an employee.

Roger believed that he was being unfairly treated and tried to fight back. He discussed the matter with the personnel manager, but was accused of using his condition to frustrate his supervisors. Finally, he was asked to leave. He requested a settlement and stood firm. He had the support of his physician, who knew of several people who had similar experiences. The reaction of the company was hostile and negative, and Roger found the personal cost of fighting for his rights as an employee high:

The negotiations continued for a period of two-and-a-half years and were extemely trying. At every instance I was exposed to criticism and pressure. It reached a point, from an emotional and psychological point of view, where I was drained. The company then introduced an early-retirement program. My lawyer thought that this program was as good as any settlement I would achieve in court, so I left the company.

After he took an early retirement, Roger started a consulting business which has been a great success. He has since been offered three senior-management positions and has encountered no negative reactions to the way in which he works. Since his experience Roger has met many people with diabetes who have been subjected to similar pressure to leave their jobs. He does not feel that people investigate all the avenues that are open to them when they are faced with questionable employment practices:

Most people just come unglued. They just don't know what to do. Most don't realize that they have rights. I have investigated it to the point where I now counsel people on their rights and what they should do. In almost every instance they don't realize what can happen until it happens to them.

It is unfortunate that such discriminatory practices are still part of the experience of some people. Having diabetes may make work life more complex, but it does not interfere with productivity.

Controlling diabetes at work

Many people did not mention having difficulties at work. They took pride from the fact that they were so healthy, as the following two quotes illustrate:

I'm a foreman. My job takes me all over the plant. I'm very active and have to contend with different things. I don't think diabetes has slowed me down. I've never missed a day's work.

I hold down a full-time job. My absentee leave has been less than my non-diabetic co-workers.

Others, however, found that mixing diabetes and work was difficult. Ellen had had diabetes for thirty-nine years. She reflected on the added demands posed by diabetes over the course of her career:

A career without diabetes would have been somewhat easier because of problems getting a job and passing medicals. It is bound to make someone insecure. Whether your employer knows about it or not, it still leaves you a little vulnerable in the workplace in terms of exertion or going on assignments. Some people handle it better than others. It does create an extra demand. You couldn't keep up in the same sense. Especially these days when the competition is so fierce. People should be able to cope with it. It's just that it's an extra thing to cope with.

Those who had difficulty talked primarily about how work affected diabetes management. The working environment was the single most important aspect that was identified as affecting diabetes control. Job-related stress and meetings were two features of work that were discussed most frequently. Although everyone faces job-related stress, it is more critical for those with diabetes because if can elevate blood glucose levels and make control more difficult. Sometimes the stress was related to the demands of the job itself, such as pressing deadlines or salary negotiations. More frequently people described stress associated with interpersonal relationships. In either case, if the stress continued at high levels for a long period of time, the solution, more often than not, was finding a different job.

Meetings were another aspect of the job that could pose difficulties. Although the impact of meetings on diabetes control was far less serious than job-related stress, it still required some effort to minimize it. The biggest problem was meetings that ran over the lunch hour. Because of not wanting to be conspicuous, people were often hesitant to suggest breaking for lunch. Some people, in fact, would not interfere with meetings and faced the risk of hypoglycemia. Others found additional ways to cope.

Craig, for example, stood his ground, and insisted on taking a break:

I used to have long sessions with the president of the company which would start at eight in the morning and end at eight in the evening. There was no food schedule. I would just get up any time in the meeting and say 'It's time for a coffee break.' I would get a scowl but I'd just say, 'You can sit around here until you're blue in the face, but I'm going to have a bun and a coffee.' Some people wouldn't know that I was a diabetic, but eventually they would find out or I'd tell them. I would say to them, 'You should all follow my example and you'll be better off than you are right now.' That was my offhand way of saying that they were crazy and I wasn't going to do it. Lunch time is twelve, not two-thirty standing around the coffee machine. I wouldn't have said it that way if I'd been under different circumstances. I could have taken more flack for it because they might have thought that I wasn't as dedicated as the rest, but I did fine. Some people think it's great when I'm around, because they always know they're going to eat on time.

Gwyn preferred a more subtle approach:

If I go into a meeting at eleven and it's still going on at two, I'll either send a note to whoever is chairing the meeting saying, 'Coffee?' or I'll get up from the table and excuse myself for a couple of minutes and take a washroom break. If I've got my sandwich with me in my purse, I will just go out and walk up and down the corridor while I eat my sandwich.

In the examples we have presented above, individuals themselves took responsibility for solving the difficulties arising because of work and diabetes. It was also evident from our conversations that other factors contributed to the ease with which people could cope effectively. One such factor is the degree of flexibility available at work. The following two examples show the significance of job flexibility:

I'm a supervisor; I can do what I want. I can stop work if I need to and have an orange at my desk. If I operated a machine, I couldn't stop the machine and eat. Even if my boss knew I was diabetic, I couldn't do that because my buddy operating the machine next to me would question why I could do that and he couldn't. If the whistle doesn't blow, I stop at three o'clock anyway and have coffee and cookies. I can do that. The hourly rated people have to keep with it if they don't get an afternoon break.

It's not a job where I have to do rotating shift work. I can take the needle at the same time in the morning and go to work at the same hour. I can take my lunch when I want to. I can eat my snack at my desk or go to the cafeteria. I keep things in my desk drawer so I have things on hand. I can test my blood at work. I've got everything at hand. This makes handling diabetes that much easier and less stressful. It's not like a job in construction where I might be on top of a building.

Another factor that eases coping is company policy on sick leaves and medical appointments. It helped when doctors' appointments were not questioned and paid sick leave was provided. A number of people were allowed sick leave to attend diabetes-education programs.

Finally, the degree of support provided by a supervisor could have a significant impact on the quality of life on the job. Allowing flexibility, particularly during the initial adjustment to diabetes, could be crucial. In Steven's case, his duties were shifted for a short time period:

My job requires a lot of travelling. My greatest concern was how to apply diabetic control to travel. I told my boss that I wanted to get used to it and learn how to handle it before I travelled overseas. I needed and was granted three months to adjust to the diet and to feel completely confident to go through different time zones.

In Carol's case, her immediate supervisor supported a creative solution to her problem:

The vision problem was terribly frustrating for me at work. I didn't want to take time off because I needed the

*money. I couldn't see so I took a magnifying glass to
work. My boss wanted to know how soon my eyes would
adjust. I said 'If I knew I'd tell you but I don't. They could
adjust in a short period or it could be several months.' He
wasn't too happy. The customers didn't mind; they
thought it was a terrific idea. There are so many middle-
aged people that have eye problems. If they asked me, I
would say that I had diabetes and it was affecting my eyes.
The assistant manager knew I needed the money. He told
the boss that he would have to be the one to tell me to
stay home because he wasn't going to do it. I guess my
boss didn't have enough guts to do it, so I worked the
whole time.*

Summary

It was encouraging to discover that in most instances work
did not pose major difficulties in adjusting to diabetes. As
with social interactions generally, the central issue was decid-
ing whether to disclose the presence of diabetes. The fear of
stereotyping was a concern, and people had to decide for
themselves how important it was to discuss with friends or
colleagues. Diabetes was not a negative influence on most
families and if it was, it usually reflected underlying problems
that were unrelated to the condition.

EXERCISES

The common denominator of the broader impact of diabetes is all the people in your life. The first exercise below can be done without particular reference to diabetes. It will then serve as background to the exercises that follow it that are more specific to diabetes. If some of the people in your life are there only because of diabetes, you may wish to note that in the first exercise.

A / The people in your life

On a sheet of paper draw a small circle in the centre and put your name on it. Then draw other circles around the first to represent the individuals or groups of people in your life. Position the circles in such a way that the space and connecting lines you next draw suggest intimacy or distance, cooperation or opposition. Include relatives, friends, work associates, and others. You may identify them with initials or symbols. When you have finished the chart of people in your life, look it over carefully. Then use a phrase or sentence to capture your reactions to it.

Next write a brief note to each person or group you identified. Say something specific to each of them about your relationship, what you would like from them, or what you want them to know. You may wish to put these aside and add to them as time goes on.

B / Telling others

Using the list you created above, examine each person or group you identified and answer the following questions:
a / Whom have you told that you have diabetes?
b / Whom would you feel comfortable telling?

c / Whom would you not feel comfortable telling?

d / Next to each person or group, write your reasons for your choice.

e / Note which category is larger – those you have told or will tell or those you haven't and won't. How do you feel about this?

f / For each group list the pros and cons of your choice.

Look back over your lists and your notes. Do you feel any differently about any of your choices? What are the trade-offs you would have to make if you want more help and support?

C / Reactions

We have seen that participants often faced a dilemma: too little or too much attention. This exercise will clarify your reactions to this sort of dilemma as you interact with people.

Rule a page with three columns headed SITUATION, THEIR REACTION, and MY REACTION. In the first column write a one-liner about some work or social situation when you felt unhappy about another's response to an incident related to diabetes. In the second column write two reactions: your fantasy of the worst possible 'too much attention' reaction and the worst possible 'too little attention' reaction. Then in column three write your own gut reactions to each. Be honest and don't spare your feelings. Just labelling your feelings is often a good thing to do.

After you repeat this process for four or five situations, review your chart. Has your attitude changed toward any situation? What would be the best possible reaction for each situation? Could you now outline a Choice A and an Option B (see 'Option B's,' page 64) to deal with these situations as effectively as possible in the future?

D / The people at work

This exercise is based on one suggested by Richard Bolles. You may find that you like or dislike some of the people you work with for general reasons, and others for reasons related to diabetes.

a / Many people love their work but dislike some of the people with whom they work. Others hate their jobs, but stay because they like the people. This exercise may help you pinpoint the important factors at your work. Make a list of *all* the words you can use to complete this sentence:

I dislike working with people who are ...

Next to these words list *all* the words that you can use to complete this sentence:

I enjoy working with people who are ...

Be sure to include general factors and factors related specifically to diabetes.

b / Since you probably have two long lists, read them over carefully and then fill out the lists below with five factors each:

I'M TURNED OFF BY   I'M MOST HAPPY
PEOPLE WHO ARE: WHEN PEOPLE ARE:

c / Look back over your final lists. How much are your feelings about the people at work related to diabetes? If diabetes plays a central role in your feelings can you identify some steps you could take to lessen its significance? If your work situation is stressful you might find it useful to repeat this exercise but substitute 'in situations that' for 'people who are.' Make this substitution in parts (a) and (b) and then answer the questions in (c).

E / **Negative feelings**

We all have feelings toward others that we don't feel good about. We often feel that someone else is making our life more difficult. This is particularly true when we are feeling stressed.

Sometimes the best way to deal with negative feelings is simply to let them out. Once released, they may well go away. Here are two ways to do that:

a / Think of a person who is making your life with diabetes more complicated or difficult. Write a description of your interactions. Allow your negative feelings to come out. Be frank. Be open. What distresses you? What makes you feel put down or inferior? Then read over your notes and try to answer some of these questions.
  - What is the overall impact of your description?
  - How do you feel about what you have written?
  - Reread the description and see if there are any positive aspects of the situation that make you feel less hostile.

b / Think of a recent situation related to diabetes where you felt frustrated and angry, or experienced other strong feelings. Write a letter to one of the people involved (you don't have to send it). Say what was on your mind in the harshest, most pungent words you can find. Don't mince your words. Overdo it if you like. When you are finished, read your letter out loud. Then write down feelings, thoughts, new ideas, or plans that come to mind.

CHAPTER SIX

Seeking help

Chapters 3 through 5 described the day-to-day lives of many of the people we interviewed. They concentrated on the difficulties they faced and the long-term process of integrating diabetes into their lives. In this chapter we will discuss the specific activities that people initiated in order to manage their lives better. We saw earlier how a lack of knowledge about diabetes created a sense of uncertainty for many people about how well they could manage. Reading books and pamphlets, discussing concerns with health professionals, and attending diabetes-education programs all helped overcome the lack of confidence that was evident initially. Frequently, however, the best help of all came from others who had diabetes. They understood, better than anyone, the ups and downs, the fears and frustrations, and the challenge of living with diabetes.

Written materials

During the early stages of diabetes reading about the condition was one thing that helped people feel more in control of the situation. Participants described reading everything they could find ranging from books, newspapers, and magazines to medical textbooks and journals. Even after they acquired an initial overview of diabetes they continued to read to keep up to date on the latest developments in diabetes care, as well as to learn new tips for coping.

The Canadian Diabetes Association (CDA) was frequently mentioned as a good source of written material. CDA publishes many informative pamphlets and their cookbook, *Choice Cooking*, was enthusiastically welcomed. Members of CDA receive newsletters and the magazine *Diabetes Dialogue*, which contains articles (some written by people with diabetes) on such topics as diet, lifestyle, and exercise, as well as reports of recent advances in diabetes research and management. Readers described it as an interesting, informative magazine that helped them learn from others' experiences and keep up to date. There is a section at the end of this book that lists the names and addresses of the local affiliates of the Canadian Diabetes Association. There is also a list of books and pamphlets that provides more information about diabetes.

Health professionals

Our participants spoke at length about their experiences with the health professionals they consulted, especially physicians. People expected their doctor to be knowledgeable and up to date about all facets of diabetes management. They appreciated physicians who took the time to answer questions in a non-patronizing manner. However, the majority of people expected, and frequently received, far more from their doctors. They wanted their views to be listened to and respected. Some believed that in terms of day-to-day management they knew more than their physicians. Many wanted physicians to recognize their expertise and their ability to manage their own diabetes care responsibly. Repeatedly, our participants stressed the degree of emotional support provided by health professionals. They needed and were given time to discuss problems in a frank and open manner. The vast majority were pleased with the medical care and the support they received. In the few cases where people were dissatisfied they changed doctors; because they lived in a large urban setting this was a relatively easy task. Making this change was seen as an important step in 'owning' personal responsibility for managing diabetes.

Following are some excerpts from our conversations with Sarah. She describes her first doctor and the difficulties she encountered. She then describes the support she received from her new doctor. Her comments capture many of the points stressed by others and clearly communicate the positive role health professionals can play in the lives of people with diabetes:

Initially I was under the care of a doctor with the golden rule that you must keep your blood sugar within normal limits. It was at a time when it was hard to control my blood sugar. I wasn't getting any help in coping. I was just told that I must be doing something wrong. I also wasn't getting any credit for having any knowledge of the disease. She wouldn't acknowledge that stress or emotional problems could be a factor in control.

I've switched to another doctor who has far more recognition of the ebb and flow. I'm fortunate to have a doctor who recognizes that I have the ability to learn. I have met other patients of hers and she will allow you to manage your diabetes to the extent that you wish to. If you wish to abdicate responsibility she'll take it for you. But if you don't she'll help you handle it as much as you can. I've gone into her office and just fallen apart and that's all right, too. The first time that happened I went in and said, 'It's not working! Nothing is working.' We sat down and systematically went through what was happening and decided to split my insulin dose. This allows me to vary my

*insulin with my lifestyle. She allows me to get out of line
without feeling that I've failed or that something is wrong
with me because I can't always keep my blood sugar in
line. It's a real partnership.*

*I've been better. My diabetes is not necessarily better,
but my feelings about it have been much better and I'm far
more optimistic about handling it.*

Diabetes-education programs

There are now diabetes-education programs in many cities
across Canada. They are usually offered by outpatient
departments of hospitals and are staffed by nurses, physicians, dietitians, and social workers. Their purpose is to teach
people about the treatment of diabetes. The programs vary,
but often teaching takes place in a group with additional time
available for individual counselling. They also vary in length
from one-day sessions for a number of weeks to programs of
one to two weeks' duration. The programs played a very
significant role in helping the people we spoke with learn
more about diabetes and how to cope with it.

Although some people attended courses immediately after
diagnosis, most were encouraged to wait a few months
before going. The soundness of this advice is evident in the
following quote from Nancy:

*My doctor sent me to the program several months after I
got diabetes. He didn't want me to go immediately. He
said to live with it for a few months until you know the
different things that are happening to you. He was right. I
felt like I was back at school. They had a dietitian, social
worker, and doctor working with you. You could ask
questions that came up in the group, like what to do if
your meal is delayed or you are eating out – problems I
would have never thought of when I wasn't diabetic.*

*Each person is an individual. The food plan they worked
out for you goes by your weight, how much insulin you
are on, and how active you are. They watch you inject
insulin to make sure you are doing it correctly. I brought
my own equipment and gave myself insulin there. They
take urine and blood tests. They gave us literature. There
was a lot of support.*

The programs were even beneficial to people like Lorraine
who had had diabetes for thirty years:

*I had never gone to anything like a diabetes-education pro-
gram. I had read and understood the basics. I was asking
my doctor a lot of questions because I wanted to do things
differently. He suggested I go. It was an opportunity for
him to have four days of blood tests, which he never had.
I was glad I went. It helped me understand the concept of
the diet. I knew but really didn't understand what I was
doing. Now I could understand and figure it out. It gave
me the tools. It solved the mystery that surrounded where
the diet came from.*

The opportunity for daily monitoring provided valuable
information to the health professionals, who could adjust
medication and suggest other changes. In this way diabetes
control could be reassessed without the disruption of a hospital admission. Attending diabetes classes at the time of a
change in treatment can make the transition easier. The
classes were instrumental in helping Ian and his wife accept a
shift from oral medication to insulin:

*The doctor told me that I had to go on insulin. He said he
wanted me to go to the education program and they would
show me how to do it. I did it there for five days. The
nurse would watch me to see if I was doing anything*

*wrong. People there were terrific. They would do any-
thing at all to help you. I was upset the first few times I
went. I said there was no way I was going to take insulin.
By the last few sessions we had I was pretty well ready to
accept insulin. We looked at it so differently from when we
first went there. The classes prepared me to do it. When
we left, we said, 'If I have to do it, I have to do it.'*

As the quotations have shown, diabetes-education programs are an excellent source of information about the
rationale for the various forms of treatment. Understanding
'why' was important to everyone, as was the practical information. Tim's response to attending his second program in
four years was typical of most:

*I thought they were very good. They taught me everything
I had to know, all the basics – the diet, testing urine, and
being in closer touch with yourself. I took the advanced
diet class. It gave me greater flexibility in choosing my
meals. I thought it was fascinating. I got good pointers on
eating out and what foods I can substitute. They taught
how to handle reactions and stress. We talked about stress.
They brought it out of you. If you don't know the basic
tools and don't have the background knowledge, you're in
trouble right from the start. The course gave me the drive
to get going and overcome a lot of the problems I was
having.*

The 'drive to get going' that Tim experienced was one of
the major benefits of participating in diabetes-education
programs. The programs ensured that adequate time was
available to cover the important content. They also understood the importance of taking diabetes seriously and of making a concerted effort to get on top of it. As the following
excerpt illustrates, the opportunity to get the condition under

control in a supervised and supportive setting established a
momentum that carried over to daily living:

I think the program was good. It made me more conscious
of the diabetes. I found that if there was any one period
where I strictly watched what I ate it was during that time.
I was monitored closely for those two weeks in my life and
I wanted to show some improvement. I took it seriously. It
demonstrated to me how much weight you can lose by
paying close attention to it. They took blood sugar three
times a day and I saw the readings go down. I was high at
the beginning and was normal at the end of the two weeks.
It helped me to stay on the diet from there on in.

Finally, diabetes-education programs established themselves
as an ongoing source of support. If individuals had questions
or ran into problems they knew there was a trustworthy
place to call to find the answers.

If your doctor does not know where you can attend a
diabetes-education program then call or write your local
branch of the Canadian Diabetes Association. The addresses
are listed at the end of this book.

Others with diabetes

Other people who have diabetes can frequently play a very
important support role. Those who are coping well are an
inspiration during times of discouragement. In the following
example we see the significance of having a role model in the
early stages of diabetes:

My grandmother had diabetes, and in some ways it helped.
I was very fond of my grandmother and at least someone
that I liked had diabetes. It's almost like a link. It helped
me to accept diabetes in some ways. She wasn't sorry for

herself. I admired her spirit, the way she was a person. I guess I thought, 'Well, if it means being like her, maybe it's not such a bad thing.'

Others described success stories – people they knew who had achieved what they sought; for example, losing weight, having healthy children, or simply coping with confidence. In contrast, there were some who saw the results of poor control in people they knew and were motivated to avoid the same mistakes.

Meeting others with diabetes to exchange information and ask questions helped our participants discover tips for coping. They shared the kinds of things health professionals would be unlikely to discuss:

I thought I was the only bad person who cheated and had sweets. I started to meet others with diabetes and learned I wasn't the only one. I thought, 'They do it too. I'm not so terrible!' They could also tell me how to make allowances for it, whereas my doctor would just say that I shouldn't do it. I was feeling there was no way around the things I was craving. Knowing that the option to cheat is there, even if I'm not sure it's worth it, helps because I feel that my life is at least partially normal.

Others with diabetes are able to lend a sympathetic ear because they have walked the same road and know its pitfalls. People were relieved to talk to someone without having to give detailed explanations:

I have found that it's very helpful to call other diabetics, not necessarily for information, but just to unload sometimes. You're perhaps having a difficult time and you want to talk it through. You don't exactly set out to do it, but you find somebody else who has also had a similar kind of problem. With most other diabetics you talk to, you don't have to explain it exactly. You sort of describe the situation and they understand. They'll listen for a while, and you'd do the same for them. I think this is particularly helpful.

Meeting others with diabetes is not always easy. It was hard to find organized support groups except in places where the Canadian Diabetes Association sponsored them. Those who had participated in such groups found them useful, particularly because they provided a forum where they could work through their own feelings and attitudes toward diabetes. Elizabeth captured the positive aspects of such groups:

I read an ad for the Adult Discussion Group in the Diabetes News. *I thought, 'This is it, this is perfect.' I went to the group and it helped. It helped to see these people and think, 'We all went through this, the shock of being told and the fears.' At least once a month you're not the exception to the rule. You are the rule. It's really good. It's emotionally and practically helpful. I was looking for support. I think I had all the facts and information I could stand. I didn't need any more. I needed somebody to talk to and say, 'Yeah, I feel the same way.'*

After twenty-eight years of belonging to a similar group, Ellen was still as enthusiastic as Elizabeth:

I have gone to a group of diabetic women for twenty-eight years. Whatever problem comes up, there's usually somebody else you can chat with – not necessarily to get direct advice, but it's often reassuring to talk about your fears or problems day-to-day when no one else has the time to listen.

A number of participants believed such groups should be readily available and were concerned that they were not. As Elizabeth said, 'When you're feeling low anyway, you don't have that much strength to really go out and search for it.' As a consequence once they felt on top of diabetes many people looked for other ways to help. Some entered health professions to put their own experience directly to work. Others did volunteer work for CDA and its affiliates. A few people expressed a specific interest in starting a self-help group but were uncertain about how to begin. For those who are interested in self-help groups, some references on setting them up have been included at the end of this book. Many participants consented to be interviewed for this book because they wanted to help others by sharing their experiences. They were certain that a major source of strength and encouragement came from firsthand experience from 'someone who knows':

The trouble is that if you haven't lived through the experience, you see the anger and you just throw up your hands and say, 'This person does not want any help,' and wash your hands clean. But if you've lived through it you know that the best thing is just to let them thrash it out. There are times when they need that. They need someone who is strong and has a certain kind of sympathy.

Gaining confidence in one's ability to cope with diabetes comes with time and experience. Actively seeking assistance can help with the hurdles. Books, health professionals, diabetes-education programs, and people who have diabetes can all help a person by providing additional knowledge, a sympathetic ear, and help with problem solving. The sense of teamwork and mutual support helps inspire confidence and competence to meet the recurring challenges.

EXERCISES

A / Assessing sources of support

To help identify your sources of help and support in coping with diabetes, consider the various people in your life; they may include family members, friends, others with diabetes, and your doctor or other health professionals. List these people down one side of a page leaving lots of room between each name. Consider the following questions for each person:
- What do they do that is helpful or supportive? If you cannot think of anything say so. What behaviour is not supportive?
- Is their support practical or emotional? For example, practical suport may be help with diet; emotional support may be listening to problems.

Given this information, check off those people in your life who play an important supportive role. What is the dominant kind of support they provide?

B / What support would you like to have?

Do this exercise in three steps:
a / If you were free to create your own supportive environment in which to cope with diabetes, what support would it provide? How would it be provided? Write down what you would really like and try to be as specific as possible. Dream a bit and ignore any possible barriers.
b / Now come back to reality. Examine the sources of support you identified above. Are the various people in your life providing the supportive behaviour you would like to get from them?
c / What kind of behaviour is not supportive? Why is it not supportive? How would you like to see it change? How can you change your reaction to it?

C / Meeting your needs for support

If your needs for certain kinds of support are not being met, how can you solve this problem?

a / The problem: First clearly state what the problem is and why it is a problem. Complete the open-ended sentences below, trying to be as specific as possible.

How to ...

This is a problem because ...

Here is an example of how to write down one problem:

How to find help and support when I'm really feeling frustrated by diabetes.

This is a problem because I find that the demands of the diabetes regimen are sometimes difficult to tolerate. I do not know of anyone who understands this and can help me deal with the times it really gets to me.

b / The solution: Write down all the solutions you can think of even if you think they are unrealistic or far-fetched. It helps to do this with a friend because he or she might help you discover a solution you would have never thought of on your own.

Here is one possible solution to the problem described above. Contact someone living in your community who has diabetes and see if she or he would be interested in getting together once in a while to share experiences.

c / Analysing the solution: Indicate what you like and do not like about each of the solutions. What are the limitations? What does it not solve? Here is an analysis for the solution above.

I like

- Someone else who has diabetes is most likely to share my frustration with diabetes.
- I would not have to explain a lot of details since they are familiar with the daily demands of diabetes.

I don't like
- I may not feel comfortable with this person because our personalities are different and this will get in the way of sharing our experiences.
- I would find it difficult to approach someone I do not know and ask if he/she would be willing to share his/her personal life with me.

d / Action plan: Once you have decided on the best possible solution write down the steps you will have to take to put it into action and the time period in which you would like to do it.

CHAPTER SEVEN

For family and friends

This chapter is written specifically for families and friends of people who have diabetes. Although you may not want to read the entire book, you might find Chapter 5 interesting. It describes how diabetes has an impact on relationships with family, friends, and colleagues.

It is not easy to generalize about the most appropriate help that can be offered to a person with diabetes. Different people have different needs or a person might have different needs at different times. The best rule of thumb is to ask what you can do to be supportive and to *listen* to the answers.

Family support

Help and support are perhaps most crucial for those who develop diabetes when they are children or young adults. Because we interviewed only adults, we do not have a lot of information about parental support. However, from talking with people who developed diabetes while living with their parents we did learn support was crucial. In ideal situations, parents provided practical help with such things as insulin injections, meal preparation, and food selection, as well as strong emotional support. Tim, who had very positive recollections of his mother's assistance, captures many of the elements of support that others described as important:

My mother knew what to say to me to try to bring my spirits up. When I couldn't find it, she gave me a brighter outlook on diabetes. She could help me see what was going on inside me. She helped me realize there was someone who really did care about me. She also looked after my diet for a good four or five years. She got me started. At first I let my mother look after me because I wasn't looking after myself. If it weren't for her I would have cheated more. I felt I had to do my part and cheating was not doing my part. She was training me for getting out on my own.

The real challenge for parents is to learn to offer support without insisting on obedience, especially once the initial learning phase is over. As the children learned to cope, the parents had to 'fade out,' as one participant said, and allow them to take over the responsibility for management. Parents needed to exercise tolerance especially when the children were testing the limits of diabetes control, but the restraint was worth it. Once a supportive relationship had been set in motion it could last a lifetime. Many people made reference to ongoing contact with a parent once they themselves had reached adulthood, during periods when managing diabetes was difficult.

For those who developed diabetes during adulthood the support of family members could be a real plus. There were many examples of situations where spouses made a deliberate effort to learn about the condition so they could be helpful. This was particularly true in more traditional families where older men relied on their wives to prepare meals. In these circumstances their wives went to classes, studied the diabetes diet, and generally supervised their husbands' eating behaviour. In other instances a spouse might either follow all or parts of the diet and provide positive reinforcement for sticking with it. Nancy's family is one example:

My husband's been very supportive by following the same diet I am. He's eating more vegetables and fruit than he did. He feels that he looks better and feels better. My children are more aware of eating nutritionally. This has made a big difference in their lives. They think about what they eat and they are aware when I discipline them as to what I can eat.

Much of the support provided by family members was moral support. Eileen saw this as the only possible kind:

The best form of help a family member can supply is emotional support. There's nothing physical that any member can do to help you. Your management is your responsibility. They understand you have needs that are different from theirs. It goes with the basic consideration of another human being. The basic underlying word is understanding. I don't see anything wrong with expecting your family to understand that.

She also believed that to be understanding it was necessary to be educated about diabetes:

I assumed my family knew as little about diabetes as I did. Their need to know isn't as great as mine, but it was important for me that they understand. I've given them information and they've asked questions. There's been a dialogue and an awareness.

Some of the people we interviewed described attitudes of spouses that helped them maintain a balanced perspective. Sam described his wife's attitude and his own reactions:

She has helped me put it into perspective. It isn't the kiss of death; it isn't the end of the world – it is only that the pancreas is not functioning 100 per cent. She says I have to recognize that anybody that gets to later middle age has some problems to contend with, whether it's high blood pressure, heart disease, arthritis, or diabetes. Whatever it is we all have some cross to bear as we grow older. She said, 'Let's not go overboard on this thing. You ought to lead a normal, active life and not behave like an invalid.' And that has been an inestimable help to me – to have that kind of reassurance.

The nature of support is not always straightforward. A number of participants stressed their need to be responsible for themselves and their resentment of any behaviours that they viewed as overprotective or overindulgent. In the following excerpt Catherine describes the importance she ascribes to self-reliance, but also acknowledges her ambivalence:

My husband deliberately hasn't changed his eating habits because of my diabetes. He feels it's healthier for me if he doesn't. It leaves me free to make my own choices. It's less parental. His way is more like treating me as if I were normal. He isn't pandering to me, babying me, There's a part of me who's very relieved about that, very glad. There's another part that asks, 'Why doesn't he help me more?' Again, there's always that ambivalence – wanting to be independent but also wanting to be dependent; wanting to take care of myself but also wanting to be taken care of.

People appreciated responses that expressed caring and understanding. As the following quote illustrates, this kind of support is what keeps people going:

What made me feel good was a note from one of my children saying that he admires my courage, the way I've handled myself since diabetes happened. This gave me more courage. My children have been marvellous, that's what keeps me going, the support of my family.

There were a few people who had never even thought about how the family might have a role in helping them:

I am independent and shy away from depending on someone. It's not that I don't want to share with others; it's just that I don't have to. I can sort of plod on my own little route. I think that's probably what I've done.

Sharing diabetes with the family? I don't think I ever thought about it. I didn't consider that this was something that should be shared. This was my domain, my daily work. I had to deal with it. I'm just not conditioned the other way.

Some people may, in fact, need very little support. Alternatively, perhaps family members were supportive in such a low key way that the individuals never noticed.

Support of friends

This section briefly discusses positive and negative responses to learning that a friend has diabetes. On the negative side – it can be upsetting when your response is overly dramatic or too serious. One of the women we interviewed described reactions that troubled her:

When people find out I have diabetes, I think they respond as well as they can, but often they'll go, 'Oh, no!' That bothers me. In the very beginning I didn't want to tell

*others because I thought they would feel sorry for me. I
don't want to be pitied. I want to be seen as in control
instead of having people feel that I'm victimized. I guess it's
my ego. I just don't want to feel that I'm the low one on
the totem pole.*

Conversely, no reaction at all was interpreted as indifference
and was also not appreciated. The best response appeared to
be a balanced one that indicated interest, curiosity, and concern. The three quotes that follow illustrate the importance of
such responses:

*When I did get up the courage to tell somebody I had dia-
betes, I was always pleasantly surprised and relieved when
they responded by saying that that was very interesting
because their aunt had diabetes, too. They were interested,
and I could teach them something about diabetes.*

*The reactions are very individual but I think there's more
caring reactions than uncaring reactions. For example, 'Oh,
you're a diabetic. How do you keep it in line?' They
express a valid sense of curiosity, but that's about as far as
it goes.*

*I was actually more than happy to explain diabetes to him
because he showed that he cared. You can almost pick up
that feeling from people who are actually really concerned
for me. It's not just their own curiosity. When somebody
does really show concern, it makes me feel good inside.*

There are times with diabetes when more than anything
else, people need an opportunity to talk. As Tim said, 'It
helps to get things off your chest.' Friends who were willing
to serve as a listening post were especially valued because it
was often difficult to find people who could empathize. Par-

ticipants were seeking understanding and sensitivity. They hoped that reaching out to friends would lessen the loneliness they sometimes felt. In the following excerpts three people described how friends could support them:

I think it would be great if people could understand diabetes and be able to help. Even if you are not a diabetic, there are things you can learn about it. It's nice to know that you are not alone in it because you know that other people understand it. I guess in a sense it's becoming sensitive to what the person is going through and the support they need from other people so that they don't leave people with diabetes off in the corner. They still should be seen as part of the society.

I would like my friends to know a bit about the disease so that they could ask me about the problems I'm having and I could share my experiences with them. It is an issue dealing with close friends, because they don't understand diabetes and I can't preach to them. I want them to understand that I've changed. My life is more prescribed, but it can be just as full.

I don't want people to feel sorry for me, yet on the other hand I don't like people to make light of it. I'd like understanding. I wouldn't want to be in my situation if I had the choice. I don't like somebody to tell me that it's not so terrible. I feel like saying to them, 'Okay, you deal with it.'

Some friends expressed support by actions other than listening. For example, Rosemary's friend bought a diabetes cook book and tried to follow along with the diet, believing it was good for her as well. Gwyn's friends helped her ignore the temptation of certain foods, reinforcing that they were not for her. Others might consider such behaviour interference, which underscores the importance of sensitivity in responding to people's individual needs.

Another area that requires sensitivity is how you handle situations that might call public attention to your friend's diabetes. The most commonly cited examples dealt with food. Several of our participants cited examples where their host prepared special food for them when they would have preferred to eat what they could from the selection of food available for others. They knew that special preparation signified a caring attitude yet they disliked being singled out for special attention. On the other hand, they were embarrassed when food was pushed on them, especially desserts. Some suggested that the best way to handle situations such as these is to either check in advance how your friend would like to handle both food selection and meal hours or to inform them privately and in advance of your planned arrangements so they can make the necessary adjustments.

Ultimately, most of the people we interviewed preferred to shoulder the responsibility for the condition. They liked to make their own decisions about how to handle management issues like food. They did not want special treatment that would call public attention to their diabetes. Nevertheless, there were times when they needed someone to talk to who could respond with empathy and understanding. Friends and family members who can do this will learn, from listening, how they can best respond to individual needs in ways which are supportive.

CHAPTER EIGHT

Control: The ultimate challenge

Introduction

In Chapters 4 through 6 of this book we have seen how people learned, on a daily basis, to live with diabetes. Chapter 4 showed the importance of learning by doing and the role of trial and error in coping with the restraints and limitations that are part of diabetes management. Chapter 5 highlighted the potential impact of the condition on one's family, social, and work lives. The nature of the interactions in these settings forced individuals to confront the attitudes of others towards diabetes. Chapter 6, which focused on help and support, illustrated the importance of enhancing and expanding on what is learned through doing, by ensuring that opportunities exist for information input and reflection with others. All of the topics described in these chapters are important facets of coping with diabetes. However, the issue most crucial to our study participants was resolving the degree to which they were prepared to allow diabetes to dominate their lives. Those individuals who appeared to have peacefully integrated diabetes into their day-to-day lives had a clear sense of how much emphasis they would place on diabetes management. The bottom line of diabetes management is control. As one participant said:

The comment the doctor made initially was one that really hit home. He said you can let it control you or you can control it. If there was a single element that made sense to me and allowed me to carry on, that was it.

Control and attitudes toward it were at the root of each individual's attempts to come to terms with diabetes and to rearrange his/her life in response to it.

It was evident from our conversations with people that the term 'control' had two meanings. First, it referred to the activities necessary for achieving the optimal level of blood glucose and included dietary restrictions, the administration of insulin, physical exercise, and the maintenance of certain routine activities and time patterns. Second, control represented the emotional and physiological mastery of diabetes in order to minimize its negative impact on a person's life. It is the second meaning that will be explored in this chapter.

The personal significance of mastering diabetes depended in part on an individual's personality. For the meticulous, self-disciplined, and cautious, mastery was often less important or irrelevant because it could be achieved with relative ease. However, those who were adventuresome, independent, unmethodical, and impulsive were quite adamant about their need to control diabetes in ways that did not compromise their personalities.

It is paradoxical that, in seeking to control diabetes, the individual must, first of all, concede that diabetes is an exacting taskmaster. To succeed at mastering diabetes one must first acknowledge its power. This recognition is frequently an integral part of coming to accept, emotionally as well as intellectually, that one has diabetes and has it for life. The challenge then is to come to peace with it.

Meeting the challenge

There were as many different stories of coming to terms with diabetes as there were people telling them. For some, the path to a harmonious coexistence was easy; for others it was long and difficult. Tim's story represents one of the more difficult experiences. Excerpts from his conversations are presented because his story clearly illustrates the struggle to master diabetes and the shifts in attitude that can be experienced during the process. Tim has had diabetes for eight years. Soon after it was diagnosed, he became frustrated with the limitations it imposed:

I thought, 'I'm going to have to live my whole life like this. I don't call this living!' I couldn't do anything I wanted because it limited me in so many different things. I felt I was always left out of something. I couldn't do things with the other guys. I just wanted to be one of them.

He then moved into a phase of denial:

I was at the stage where I wanted to ignore the whole situation. I didn't want to think about it. I didn't want to talk about it. I didn't want anything to do with it because it was upsetting. I just wanted to get on with my life. I didn't want to hear about diabetes. I felt like it was taking priority over everything and why should I let it. So I thought, 'I'm not going to let it run me. I'm going to put diabetes near the bottom of the list.'

However, relegating diabetes to the bottom of the list was not the solution to Tim's problems:

I couldn't bury it because it was with me twenty-four hours a day. My sugar was going up. I was losing weight. My life was a mess.

Tim was forced to reevaluate:

I decided I had to do something or I'd never get out of the rut I was in. I had to get a new attitude or else I wasn't long for this world. That's what triggered it. I just came to the realization that I had to act because if I didn't, something was going to happen to me and I'd wish I'd never lived as I had. So I thought, 'Why not at least try to fight it and smarten up?' I decided I would try accepting it. It seemed a little easier when I did that. I faced up to what could really happen to me and became aware of what I was doing instead of ignoring it and paying for it in the end.

Tim spoke to his doctor and enrolled in a diabetes-education program. He shifted his emphasis to 'self-discipline' and 'responsibility.' His goal became 'conquering diabetes.' In retrospect, Tim thinks he succeeded:

I've had diabetes for eight and a half years and I've gone through some changes and I've mastered it pretty well. It hasn't stopped me from doing too many things.

Diabetes is a really tough thing to master but it can be mastered. You gotta go at it full force. Facing up to it – that's the hardest part. I have to take one day at a time. If diabetes gets the better of me sometimes – fine. I'll get it more times than it gets me. I have to take my lumps. It's a personal battle that never stops. You always know when you score a victory, and it always helps make you stronger the next time. It's quite a challenge – it really is!

The battle for control

Many people we spoke to described living with diabetes as a challenge. In fact, when we examined our participants' choice of words we noted that often they were words associated with war. For these people, engaging with diabetes was a form of combat. They referred to diabetes as the 'adversary' and the 'enemy' and spoke of 'doing battle,' of 'refusing to be defeated,' and of 'conquering' and 'winning.' Comments such as the following are typical:

If you don't control it, it's going to control you. It's like a continuous challenge, day in and day out. There's not one day you get a break, not one day. You just battle it out. You take one day at a time. It's a real challenge, and if you beat it, it makes you stronger. You have to fight. If you don't it's going to defeat you. It's as simple as that. You're taking your life in your own hands. It's almost like an evil thing you've got on your back that you're trying to fight off. You've really got to stand up to it.

I am convinced that diabetes is my firing squad. It has control over my life to the degree that it is even going to decide my death.

I wondered, 'Who's going to win this war?' Well, I'm going to beat this, but at my own pace. There's no way this is going to flatten me. I'm going to pick myself up by the bootstraps and go.

Diabetes is the enemy. It can't become a friend! Ever! It's warfare, but you are at war with yourself.

Accepting diabetes

A crucial first step in the war with diabetes is learning to accept that you have it. Many people saw this as a major obstacle that had to be overcome:

You've got to deal with having diabetes. Then it becomes a lot easier. It's a mental thing. I suppose it's like beating alcoholism. The biggest thing is recognizing you have it. You have it, and no wishing can change that.

Accepting it is not saying 'I love it! I'm glad I've got diabetes.' That's not what I mean by accepting it. I hate it! I could do better without it! But I have to accept it to the point where I have to realize what it is and what it's going to do to me and that I've got to control it. It's part of me like the colour of my hair and my eyes. It's part of my physical makeup – height, weight, diabetes.

Unfortunately, acceptance does not always come easily. It may take time to recover from the shock of diagnosis:

The biggest thing was to accept the fact that I've go it, so then what do I do with it. I think it took a good six months before I could finally say, 'Okay, I can live with it.' It's something that takes time to learn. Now, after three years, I think about it only half of the time.

It can hit like a ton of bricks and turn life around completely if you let it. It does, at least at the beginning. I found the beginning difficult. I had to work at it. Now it's just an everyday type of thing that I accept. I just know I have to do these things.

Some people never really accept diabetes. Catherine, who has had diabetes for twenty-four years and who leads a full life, is one example:

I truly don't know if I will ever accept diabetes. On a functional level my behaviour indicates that I accept diabetes pretty well. I take insulin three, sometimes four, times per day. I eat according to plan, probably 90 to 95 per cent of the time. On an emotional level, what accepting diabetes means is accepting imperfection. It also means allowing diabetes to become a part of me. I just don't think it's ever going to be possible to completely accept diabetes. If diabetes becomes a part of me, at a very deep level, it would take me over because it's so powerful. It would obliterate me.

Eleanor, too, could not really accept diabetes, even though she had had it for sixteen years. And, unlike Catherine, she could not manage to follow a diabetic regimen. When we interviewed Eleanor about her life with diabetes, her anger and discouragement were frequently accompanied by tears:

I hate having diabetes, and I think it's terrible. I don't do what I'm supposed to do, and I hate all the stuff I'm supposed to do. I know what I'm supposed to do, but I don't do it. You know the stages of dying? I think this relates because I sort of look at diabetes as a terminal illness. I figure its going to kill me! I think I'm denying it; pretending I don't have it. Except, I know what I'm doing, I know I'm denying it.

Redefining control

Part of accepting diabetes is acknowledging the control it exerts particularly when it is ignored rather than respected. Catherine described the impact of this awareness on her:

My life is literally dependent on factors outside of my own will, my strength, or my ingenuity. I have difficulty accepting that I'm not powerful enough to control all the factors that influence my metabolism. It's a helpless feeling. I have wanted to control everything.

Once people acknowledged and accepted the inherent power of diabetes they shifted the focus of control from the disease to themselves. In recognizing their own potential for positive action they transformed their vision of themselves from victim to agent. Instead of representing imposed limitations and sacrifices, control became an empowering mechanism whereby people asserted their will to live a full and rewarding life within the boundaries of diabetes. Gwyn captured this idea when she said:

Diabetes is something that comes as a result of something you have no control over. But then your control is in the fact that you can do something. There are some things you can do about diabetes. You play some part in this.

Accepting the responsibility

Part and parcel of accepting diabetes and redefining control is accepting the responsibility for taking care of oneself. There was a general agreement among people about the need to 'take care':

You have to have self-discipline when you are a diabetic. Control is the most important thing. You are taking care of yourself so the responsibility has to be with you. I realized when I became diabetic that it was my responsibility.

With diabetes you have to be a responsible person. You are afflicted. It's not like an appendix that can come out. You're going to have it the rest of your life – like it or not. If you don't know what's going on with you, what are you going to do at 6 a.m. when you're throwing up, losing everything from both ends, dehydrated, and the doctor isn't there? You have to know what to do and be responsible enough to carry on a normal life.

I think when you're a diabetic you've got to deal with life as well as you possibly can. And I think that's maybe the difference. If you're not dealing with it well you better find out how to deal with it. The really important thing for me is to be well connected with life, to get pleasure out of life, because I can't indulge myself in drowning my sorrows by eating, by smoking, or by drinking. So I better bloody well have my life in order to get enough other kinds of pleasure. Developing responsibility as a diabetic cannot be divorced from one's ability to be responsible in one's life generally.

Finding a balance – the key to control

Living with diabetes – that's the best way to state the case – is living with it. Existing with it isn't worth a damn.

Living versus existing was the way many people described the challenge of diabetes. The crucial difference between 'living' and 'existing' lies in the degree of energy for and active involvement in daily life. The challenge for people with diabetes was in the struggle to live in such a way that they kept the diabetes under control without having to make major concessions to their preferred ways of living. To live well with diabetes, individuals tried to achieve 'balance.' They expressed the concern that diabetes not become 'the be-all and the end-all.' Balance, which is individually determined, describes the equilibrium that individuals achieve between their own needs and the demands of the condition. It represents, ultimately, the place of diabetes in a person's life.

The range of individual balance points can be plotted on a continuum that reflects the ease with which people can make the lifestyle changes necessary to maintain their definition of optimal control.* Generally speaking, those who found that the changes came relatively easily were those who had the fewest changes to make.

Although there was a wide range of balance points individuals tended to cluster at four points along the continuum (see Figure 1). Personality traits and the severity of the diabetes were both important factors influencing where people fit. We will use examples drawn from our interviews to illustrate these four points and the factors that influenced the ease of adjustment.

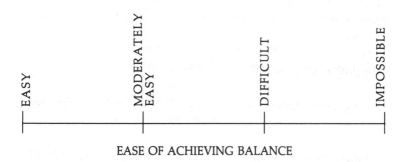

EASE OF ACHIEVING BALANCE

Figure 1 – The Balance Continuum

Easy

For those at one end of the balance continuum the demands of the diabetes regimen were not particularly intrusive. In Matthew's case, adjusting to diabetes was easy. He observed that his personality probably contributed to the ease with which he adjusted:

---

* Individual standards for optimal control might be different from medical standards.

I don't seem to have any problems with diabetes. I try to keep to the routine, and I don't do things on an ad hoc basis. I think the regimen is good for you – it's clean living. I tend to be a cautious person. I tend to think in terms of consequences. I tend to believe a lot of what I read. The authorities have told you the proper things to do to minimize complications, so I do them. I accept the authoritative view. I think the self-discipline has to come from yourself.

In Jeff's case as well, balance came easily:

I am a diabetic and nothing is going to change that. Diabetes is a part of life, an important part. If I want to continue with my life, I have to control my life. That's not as hard as it sounds. I am active. I get lots of exercise. I play ball. I do everything that every other normal person does. So I do a little more: I take an insulin shot; I'm a little more aware of my food intake. That's all right. It's become part of my life. It's important to me, but it's not the be-all and the end-all. It's just another part of your life – like going to work in the morning.

Matthew and Jeff have both been able to integrate diabetes into their lives with few compromises. Their personalities and their lifestyles were conducive to the routine and self-discipline necessary for good control.

Moderately easy

For Sarah and Craig, it was important to live in a way that allowed for flexibility and adventure. Sarah explained:

Compliance has never been easy for me – with the diet or in doing what's best for myself. A lot of people think it should be natural for me because I know and understand the consequences. It's not easier for me than for anybody else. You try to set up a routine for yourself. If you have to restrict your life too much to make that routine work, then I personally can't accept being restricted to that extent. I think at this point in my life I have recognized that, so I'm not a model diabetic patient. I'm active in my life and I don't feel restricted in anything I want to do and I don't think I jeopardize myself. But I'm not going to miss out on anything because I am a diabetic. I'm not going to stop trying out new things, some of which work and some of which don't. Restricting my lifestyle to that extent is just unacceptable. While it's an oversimplification, the simplest way of putting it is I am more concerned about the quality of my life now than I am about living to seventy.

Craig, too, elected to exercise some degree of latitude in his approach to diabetes:

You have to pick a path you can manage. I realized at some point that I'm not going to be supergood because that's not the nature of the beast, but I will certainly not be a bad or sloppy diabetic because that's not the nature of the beast either. I can't think of anything that I wanted to do or tried to do that I haven't. I work, I travel extensively, which means I eat meals in hotels. The way I live isn't very conducive to a diabetic regimen but I've done it for thirteen years.

People like Sarah and Craig were conscious of limitations and were determined to prevent these limits from taking over their lives. While they accepted some of the limitations, both of them made a deliberate effort to keep them in perspective so that the restrictions did not play a disproportionate role in their lives. While they were concerned about maintaining physiological control, they were also concerned about trying to maintain a normal life and minimizing the degree to which diabetes interfered with this goal.

Difficult

When people had a form of diabetes that was amenable to a somewhat flexible lifestyle, it was easier to be adamant about not letting it become overly intrusive. But those individuals whose diabetes was unstable were forced to live with more constraints and had to accept the fact that diabetes did dictate a certain way of life. These people simply had to make changes and adapt to a new way of living. For example, to keep her diabetes under the degree of control she viewed as necessary, Eileen governed the time frames by which she lives. She eats three meals a day at set times and three snacks a day at set times, all consisting of certain categories of food. She will not eat away from home unless she is certain that she can eat exactly at her meal time. At home she eats at five o'clock, and family members eat as they arrive. As a consequence, diabetes has compromised almost everything Eileen has wanted to do. Nonetheless, she has not felt defeated by diabetes, but has instead focused on 'positive thinking' because she feels that outlook has a very great effect on well-being. Although the regimentation in her life was a source of frustration, Eileen has persevered because her first priority is her wish to live a long life.

Roger, too, eventually made major shifts in his lifestyle. He was forced to make changes because of the impact of uncontrolled diabetes on his daily life. Ultimately, Roger viewed these changes as overwhelmingly beneficial and, as a result, changed his lifestyle values quite radically. Roger described his early years with diabetes:

I was down to 125 pounds. I had absolutely no energy. I would come home and sleep before dinner. I had lost all

*emotion. I was coming home and avoiding people because
of the possible stress situations that could occur. I would
shrink every time the phone rang. For a period of four to
five years I withdrew from social activities and community
service. Before I developed diabetes I was involved with
eleven or twelve charitable organizations. As my condition
worsened, I gave up one activity after another and got
down to zero. I had just reached the point where I didn't
have sufficient strength to have a positive outlook. I
reached the point where, in utter desperation, I felt
I simply had to do something. I just felt there was so much
I wanted to accomplish that I had to make a basic decision
on my health and where my priorities were. I decided that
I would seek assistance and comply completely with it.*

The changes Roger made in his life were significant. They
included a major career shift, serious devotion to an artistic
hobby in preparation for retirement, new choices of volunteer work, and major positive shifts in his eating, drinking,
and exercise patterns. The overall tone of Roger's conversations was one of a man who was experiencing a renewed
vitality as a result of finding a new sense of purpose in life.

Impossible

The point at the far right of the continuum represents a situation where balance is impossible to achieve because the goal
that is sought is perfect behaviour in order to achieve perfect
diabetes control. Individuals will never be able to achieve
balance if they remain obsessed with perfection, since they
must deny their personal needs and give in to the condition.
Furthermore, given the unpredictable nature of diabetes, 100
per cent perfect control is currently impossible. Catherine is
an example of a person who, at the present time, can be
found at this position on the contiuum. At first glance, she

could be included in the examples with Sarah and Craig. She values flexibility and spontaneity and has found ways to allow for them without seriously compromising her control. She could be considered a good role model because of the balance she portrays. Despite her success with coping, Catherine is not satisfied. She feels very strongly that diabetes dominates her. She characterized it as an overpowering adversary who has the power to obliterate her. She believed it had encroached on her sense of self because it implies imperfection and damage. As a consequence, Catherine viewed her attempts to coexist with diabetes as a life and death struggle, one which ultimately she cannot win. She chastised herself for fighting to satisfy her other needs, which she labelled 'indulgences.' It was a struggle to give in to her 'desires,' and she found she 'hated' herself for her 'lack of control.' Catherine was aware of the pitfalls of the trap she was in but felt powerless to extricate herself. She spoke poignantly about her struggle to be a perfectionist in the handling of diabetes:

Someday I have got to let go of my wish for perfection. I just have to lighten up on myself. The consequences are that for twenty-four years I have felt like a failure with diabetes. I continue, every day, to feel that I am failing. I have fallen from perfection. I have not achieved the ideals that I want to. When I hear that normal blood sugars can prevent complications, then I want that. That's my rosy path. Why can't I do it? Somebody must be achieving them. Why can't I? It contributes to the sense that perfect control is not an impossible task. It's just that I'm failing.

Catherine was not the only person we spoke to who struggled with perfection. Lorraine at one time had experienced similar feelings, but had moved closer to finding a balance that was more personally satisfying:

As I get older, I've discovered a lot of things are not important. I used to be more of a perfectionist than now. I've come to the realization that nobody is perfect. You can fool yourself for a long time. It's an unattainable goal, a waste of time and energy.

There is this ideal diabetic lifestyle that I resent and find I don't want to live with. You assume a certain amount of responsibility for caring about yourself and keeping healthy. But what happens if you're absolutely careful and things still go wrong?

The search for perfection is probably a hang-up. People that I know that manage perfectly have my admiration. I might feel guilty that I don't, but I know that's not a lifestyle I can follow. It's not my personality.

Lack of balance

Some of the people we talked to had not yet discovered what balance point was appropriate for them or how to achieve it. Will, for example, has had diabetes for two years. At the time he was interviewed his diabetes was not yet under control and was demanding an excessive amount of attention. He resented its intrusion into his life and longed for but could not achieve a degree of balance:

I want to be unencumbered. I want to live life in spite of, or coexist with diabetes, but I don't want to let it dominate. I've got the order in my life, but balance hasn't followed order. That's my greatest frustration. I'm doing all the right things and not seeing some profit. Everything's still in the red side of the ledger. When do I have time to do things that are significant? I want to get on with the joy of living. I have things in my life that occupy my time. My anguish comes from having to break into that time to deal with the disease. That has become the priority. The pans of the scale are not balancing, and that's what I'm looking for.

We hope, that Will, with time, will find the balance he seeks. It is probable that he will fit somewhere between the moderate and major adjustment on the balance continuum.

Summary

Whether or not their lives could ultimately be considered normal, people with diabetes were forced to face the challenge of control. The challenge was more easily met if they had come to accept diabetes as a given in their lives and hence to accept the responsibility for controlling it. The task was then to find a balance that reflected the needs dictated by their individual personalities and those dictated by their particular form of diabetes. In the final analysis, the appropriateness of the balance achieved became a judgment call that could only be truly assessed personally by the individual who had to live day-to-day with diabetes.

This chapter has described the process by which individuals integrated diabetes into their lives. Integration occurs when people find a comfortable balance between the demands of diabetes and their own personal needs. It frequently necessitates compromises to both the quality of diabetes control and preferred lifestyles but results in a state of affairs that is satisfying. Integration is the culmination of a learning process that begins when diabetes is diagnosed. Acceptance of diabetes is usually a crucial step in the process and is one which can take years to achieve. For some, coping with diabetes can feel like waging a war, albeit a strange sort of war. For before diabetes can be mastered people have to recognize that it always has the power to defeat them if they do not acknowledge it. Once acknowledged, the hostilities can be set aside and the task of integrating diabetes into the larger framework of one's life can proceed. It was quite clear from our interviews that there are many roads to integration and that the difficulty of the journey depends in part on the severity of the diabetes and in part upon one's own personality. The journey is never over. People recognize that a place that seemed satisfactory today might not feel the same tomorrow. However, on this journey our participants acquired the insights, skills, and confidence to continue their exploration and maintain the balance they always must seek.

EXERCISES

As we have just seen, the demands of life with diabetes may be very difficult to accept, since they bring you into conflict with values that are important to you. Catherine found diabetes hard to accept because she valued perfection and independence. To Sarah, flexibility and freedom were more important values than perfect control of diabetes. An important insight that our participants acquired was the understanding of values that affected their choices.

Values are deeply ingrained beliefs that determine how we act. We discover values by examining our actions, particularly consistent patterns of action. Often what we say about our values is not so important as what we actually do.

The exercises in this section are in three parts. Those in Part 1 are intended to reveal your patterns of action. In Part 2, your patterns are examined to determine the values you hold. In Part 3, these actions and values are connected to the control of diabetes. The exercises are designed for use over a few weeks or a few months. During that time you will create a lot of information about yourself. Don't throw it away. You will be able to use it over and over as time goes on.

A / Your actions

These exercises are adapted from ones suggested by Sidney Simon in his book *Meeting Yourself Halfway*.*

---

* For information about current Values Realization materials and a schedule of nation-wide training workshops, contact Sidney B. Simon, Old Mountain Road, Hadley, MA 01035, USA.

1 / Circle of life

Draw a circle on a piece of paper. Divide the circle into blocks of time to represent how you spend a typical day. Estimate the number of hours or part-hours you spend on the following activities:
- sleeping
- working at work
- working at home
- alone watching TV, reading, going to movies, other leisure activities
- with family
- with friends
- other activities (identify)
- household chores
- eating

Now divide up the circle to show how you allot your time. You may want to do other circles for a week or month. You may want to do a circle just for work or just for leisure. You could also use a circle to assess the money you spend, the kinds of shows you see, or how you feel about your day or week (good time, bad time, in-between).

After doing this circle activity several times, ask yourself these questions:
- Would I like to change the size of the slices of time?
- What would my perfect circle look like?
- What can I do to change the size of some of my slices?

Save your notes on these questions for later reference.

2 / Scenarios

Participants in our study were often confronted with hard choices. Below are two scenarios that illustrate the type of choices they had to make – read them over and then look at the instructions below. Sarah valued flexibility and freedom

more than perfect control of diabetes. She was invited to dine out. She was offered a rather exotic dish and did not know what was in it. What should she do?
- Take some but not eat it?
- Refuse it since it might upset her control?
- Accept a helping and try it out?
    Sarah did not want to miss out on anything, so she tried it. Craig travels extensively. When it comes to meals he:
- packs a lunch
- eats in hotels
- eats meals prepared especially for people with diabetes.
Craig chose to eat in hotels.
You have to make decisions like these every day, around diet, activity, social situations, and economic matters (shall I change jobs?). Write out brief scenarios like the ones here and create distinct choices. Rank the choices you would make, first, second, and third. You may draw upon actual situations you have faced. Keep track of choices you have to make. What other options did you have? If you have a friend or family member who is willing, defend your choices and discuss what others you might consider.
    Don't throw these materials away. You may wish to refer to them again.

3 / Diaries

Keep track of some specific aspects of your life. For example, you may have daily frustrations associated with diabetes. Keep notes on them for a week or a month. You may have times when you feel good about yourself over some action or decision. Keep an 'I felt good about myself' diary. You can do this for successes, good days, conflicts, or any number of other ideas. After two weeks or so review your diary and ask yourself some summary questions:
- What kinds of things frustrate me?

- What is my usual reaction? Is there a pattern?
- What do I do to blow off steam? Do I hold it in?

OR

- How often do I feel good about myself?
- What kinds of activities/discussions, etc., make me feel good?
- What rewards do I give myself?
- Do I share my good feelings with others?

When you feel you are no longer getting new ideas from one kind of diary, shift to another. Hang on to your diaries for further use.

4 / Important thoughts

Keep a diary of important thoughts every day or two, or three times a week. If possible find a friend or family member who will do the same. Every two weeks or so, sit down and share your thoughts. Ask each other these questions:
- Which of these statements represent strong beliefs that you stand for?
- Which of these statements would you change now?
- What patterns can you detect in your own thoughts or your partner's?
- Have you done anything about these strong beliefs?

After a few months try to summarize your thoughts and your discussions:
- What things interest me the most?
- How do I view my life?
- What goals do I have, short and long term?
- What are my problems, or conflicts?
- What things do I value most?

Keep your daily entries and your summaries for further reference. The materials and ideas you have collected will be useful as you move on to the next section.

B / Your values

By this time, you may already see some of your patterns of actions and the deeply ingrained beliefs they represent. Here are three ways to pin them down more closely.

1 / Priorities

Write down the people, the qualities, or ideas that are important to you. Your list might include some of these words. Don't stop until you have ten to fifteen words or phrases:

family	health	flexibility
intimacy	self-control	respect
money	independence	physical exercise

Rearrange your list into three equal sections: most important to me, least important to me, middle importance.

2 / What I say/what I do

Make two lists:
(1) What I say is important to me (2) What my actions say is important to me
Identify what items are on both lists.

3 / Learning

Complete the sections below in as many ways as seems helpful, or make up some for yourself:

I learned that _____

I was surprised that _____

I enjoyed _____

I never knew _____

c / Your values and diabetes

Here is where you connect your values with the demands of diabetes. You may find that the conflicts are familiar. Perhaps you may find some new insight.

a / Conflict: List the values and issues important to you that cause problems in controlling diabetes. Write brief comments next to each to remind you of the problems and specific details.

b / Strategies: What kinds of things have you done about each issue/value over the past one to five years (go back far enough to find a pattern if you can).

c / Patterns: List the trends or patterns for each issue/value.

d / Impact: What will happen to you (or what *does* happen to you), if you do not change this pattern.

e / Circumstances: List any circumstances that have an impact on your pattern (check back to the conflicts list).

f / Choices: At this point, you might want to redraft your list into two categories:

Things I choose to change   Things I choose not to change

g / Reframing: You can also divide your second category into two by choosing to change your feelings about this situation. One section would consist of things I choose not to change but I can change how I feel about or react to them.

d / Summary

These exercises have introduced you to identifying what you do and the values your actions represent. You may have discovered how these values conflict with controlling diabetes. There are many more exercises aimed at discovering your values and how they affect your actions. Sidney Simon's book *Meeting Yourself Halfway* is an excellent source. Very often the use of diaries and journals will extend the information you have to work with. *Keeping Your Personal Journal* by George F. Simons is a good source for that topic. Once you start on this kind of activity, it can become a lifelong tool for self-understanding. Good luck with your journey.

CHAPTER NINE

When all is said and done: Feelings about diabetes

The chronic nature of diabetes means that its demands continue over a lifetime. Many of our participants felt resentment that never disappeared. They continued to feel frustration about the limits imposed by diabetes:

It's the idea of being tied to a system – the regimentation, the bottle, the needle, and the things that surround it. It's always a constraint. I guess it's like a dog in the backyard on a rope. It must bug the dog that he's only good for six or twelve feet. Dogs don't like to be on twelve foot ropes. They like to go and run around and have a good time. And so do people. I would say that if there's one simple point to make it is the confinement or the restrictions or the limits that are hard.

I have always wanted to do a lot of things. If anything that feeling may be more pronounced now. The statistics say that because I have diabetes fifteen years of my life have been taken away from me. I keep thinking that I only have twenty-five years left and I have all these things I want to do. It has created added pressure to move that much faster. When I am reminded that my years are numbered, I feel frustrated.

In the period following diagnosis people often felt anger about having the condition. Although these feelings receded over time they did not necessarily disappear. The metaphor Lydia uses in the following quotation captures the swing in feelings that continues to occur:

It's like a fire. You get a fire going and it's blazing and then, when the flames cool down, you still have the hot ashes. You've got to be very careful, because the hot ashes can erupt. So after the anger and the thrashing and getting through all that, I said 'Okay, kid, you've got it and until they come up with a cure you're going to have it.' Occasionally you get a roaring fire again. So you've got to be careful when they are smouldering. I'm not saying that everything's completely hunky-dory. I get frustrated, but I know I have it and I'm going to have it till they come up with the cure.

Inevitably, people compared their own situation with others'. Some admitted feelings of jealousy. Tim spoke for others when he said:

I have my health, but it's not the way I would like it to be. I look at other people and I have a jealous feeling. I don't hate them; I just envy them. They don't have to worry about reactions, eating at a certain time, the needle, or getting up in the morning. On weekends they can sleep in. They don't have that extra burden on their backs in life. If I didn't have diabetes, how would life be different? I look at other people and think, 'Gee, it must be nice to have a big hunk of cake without worrying about anything except the calories.' It makes me almost hate diabetes. I think, 'Why can't I be like them? Why can't I be what they call normal?'

The tendency toward both self-pity and depression was frequently discussed. Many people experienced such feelings, but tried hard to avoid them, by keeping a perspective on diabetes. A number of people expressed the view that many worse things could happen to them. The following comments illustrate these attitudes:

I compare myself to my sister who has multiple sclerosis and I think I got off lightly. I also have a father badly crippled with arthritis, so I have a lot of comparative examples to make me feel better.

I was at a wedding last week, and of the five women at my table two had had mastectomies. I thought, 'How do I thank God that I didn't have one and how do I thank God that I'm just a diabetic?' Life falls into perspective, and you fall into perspective with that. You hear about people in such God-awful situations and then you think, 'Geez, this isn't terrific. But when you look at it relative to something like that it's really not so terrible. It's manageable.'

However, for one individual this strategy was unsuccessful and irritating:

Diabetes and cancer are the same sort of thing. Nobody wants to have diabetes. It's a very optimistic way of looking at it to say, 'Well, it's better than having cancer.' I mean it doesn't make it any easier. There's always someone worse off than you. In fact I think it really bothers me when people say, 'It's not so bad. It could be worse.' Of course it could be worse, but it doesn't mean it's not so bad.

Still, many resisted the temptation to feel sorry for themselves because, although self-pity could be comforting, they saw it as a luxury they could ill afford:

It gets to you once in a while. You say, 'Just take it away for a year. Let me have something normal.' I don't like to think this way. I can get wrapped up in the luxury of self-pity, and I cannot afford it.

The nature of diabetes caused some people to examine their lives and assess their priorities. Frequently, the daily irritants encountered in managing diabetes diminished in importance as a result. What remained was the ability to respond more positively to diabetes and its implications. One such positive response was related to a reverence for life. Not surprisingly, having diabetes often reminded the people interviewed of their mortality:

I feel very vulnerable and mortal. I feel that life is a gift and that I need to enjoy what I have while I have it, because I can't count on the future. It isn't guaranteed.

The dependence on a daily dose of insulin reinforced for Tim the fragility of life which led, in turn, to an appreciation for what he had:

I have to take one day at a time. I don't even think three days ahead. I just think only of today and then tomorrow I'll wake up and it's a brand new day and another needle. The insulin lasts twenty-four hours, so you've got another day ahead of you. Because of diabetes I have gotten closer to my inner feelings, my thinking on what issues are important to me, principles of life in general. Diabetes has changed my whole outlook on life. I guess I have learned to appreciate life more because I know I am coping with something that could kill me if I don't handle it. What's changed me is that every day I put a needle in me and I no longer take each day for granted. I appreciate every day I make it through. I appreciate the fact that tomorrow I can take the needle and it's going to allow me to ride my ten-speed bike for the day.

This enhanced awareness often served as a source of motivation for people:

My value for life has been heightened. My attitudes toward the important things of life have changed dramatically. I don't want my body to go haywire because of mismanagement. I want to live a valued, full life. I want to live long and see my children grow and see their children established in their lives. I have a lot to live for. I have a strong will to live, and maybe that is part of my motivation.

There were other positive responses to diabetes as well. Tim recognized that diabetes gave him an inner strength. As we have seen, his feelings have not always been positive. His comments revealed a very real ambivalence about the condition. Nonetheless, for Tim, the struggle to conquer diabetes has brought a sense of accomplishment and self-confidence:

I can say that diabetes has made me a better person. It's weird. I almost feel like I contradict myself when I say that because I hate diabetes, yet diabetes has made me a stronger person. It really has. The more that I think about it the more I see that it strengthened me. I do have my rough times, but I feel there are so many more good times that they wiped the rough times out. It's a day-to-day thing. It's a stupid thing to say that it's a blessing to have it but, looking back, my diabetes got me started. It made me strive to keep myself in good shape, to look after myself better. Since I got diabetes things have really picked up for me. Diabetes has done so many things to me. I used to be on the shy side and now I'm not. I feel more confident in myself. It has strengthened me.

Sarah also felt that diabetes had some very positive results for her. Like Tim, Sarah viewed diabetes as a test of her mettle:

I see the diabetes as being something that has forced me to confront certain things. You don't find out what you're really made of unless you are tested.

She identified what she saw as positive changes:

I know I'm better organized as a result of diabetes, because I have to be – not only better organized to deal with diabetes but all around. There're certain things I have to do and that spills over into the rest of my life. I tend to think ahead a lot more than a lot of people, because I can't get caught in situations I can't handle. In a way, when I look at my life, there's positive things that balance out – like the organization, the diet – you have an extra incentive to eat well; also tuning into your own body. So I don't see it all as negative.

Sarah underscored her feelings about diabetes when she said:

If I were given a chance to change one thing in my life and only one thing I can tell you right now that I wouldn't waste that chance on diabetes. I've never said that before but, in saying it now, I know absolutely that it's true.

Lynn was adamant that diabetes changed her life for the better:

I think it's changed my life a great deal because I've been forced to confront things I wasn't facing before. I think my

*life in many ways is much better now. In fact now that I'm
diabetic I don't think I'd ever want to give it up. I'm just
so much more energetic than I've been in my life before.*

Positive thinking was a part of the coping process and
Nancy is someone who was determined to think that way.
Soon after she was diagnosed, she became active in the
Canadian Diabetes Association:

*I've always had a positive attitude as far as life is con-
cerned. I try to take the good out of everything. I was put
here for a purpose. Maybe this is what I was put here for –
to be able to do something with the diabetes hitting me. I
can help people. It was a challenge to get involved with the
CDA and help others.*

Eileen found that over the course of diabetes her values
changed:

*You learn to be grateful. You learn to appreciate differ-
ently. You have a heightened awareness of things that are
good and you try to deal with the things that are negative
in your life with a different perspective. You don't dwell
on them as much. Because your energies get depleted, you
try to concentrate them where they'll do the most benefit.
Otherwise there's no purpose.*

Lydia arrived at a point that might very well be the goal of
anyone with diabetes:

*I have a sense of having come to peace with my diabetes. I
feel some sort of contentment. I think that has added to
my sense of self-confidence. I feel now that I can do anything that I wish to put my hands on. There's a contentment about not having to think about diabetes any more,
because it's a part of my life.*

'Peace,' 'contentment,' 'self-confidence,' and 'a part of my life' signify important milestones on this journey with diabetes. Lydia and many of the others who spoke with us felt they had arrived at a very satisfactory destination. They knew that circumstances would change and new challenges would emerge but they could anticipate them with the confidence of seasoned travellers. They had survived the shock of diagnosis and by taking life one day at a time had sorted out the impact diabetes would have on them. They had learned the nitty-gritty details of diabetes management and had experimented with medical guidelines to determine the limits of diabetes control. They grappled with feelings of anger, frustration, and self-pity, and overcame them. They accepted that they had diabetes and developed the will to master it. Ultimately, most people sought and achieved a degree of balance. They learned how to keep diabetes in control and to live a life that was full and satisfactory. Diabetes fell into place. It became one more facet of people's lives rather than the central focus. Its mastery brought with it a sense of accomplishment and an appreciation of life.

We hope that those of you who have recently discovered that you have diabetes will approach the challenge with optimism. Those of you who have had it longer have probably recognized many of your own experiences in the vignettes we have presented. We hope you have found the motivation to 'keep on truckin'. We wish you well!

EXERCISES

The exercises in this section are adapted from ones discussed by George F. Simons in his book *Keeping Your Personal Journal* (© Paulist Press). They are designed to help you express and assess your feelings about diabetes and to develop an image of your future.

A / We/they: Alone

Participants in our survey often spoke of feeling different from people who do not have diabetes. Sometimes they were envious of others who seemed more fortunate; at times they felt lucky compared to others who were far worse off.

Make a list of we/they's for yourself. List specific individuals and where possible, specific incidents. Describe those incidents and your feelings.

Tim (on page 138) described his we/they:

WE	THEY
I can't be normal.	They can.
I worry about reactions.	They don't.
I can't sleep in.	They can sleep in.
I can't have cake.	They can.
I have extra burdens.	They don't.

After you make your list, look back over it. Are any of your we/they's no longer relevant? Which ones are most recent? Make notes about the old ones and the new ones. Write down the impact these have on your life. Then make a new list that emphasizes what is positive in your life compared to others. Look for some 'positives' associated with diabetes.

B / We/they: With others

If you have the opportunity to work with other people in a

group setting, the we/they exercise can be even more effective.

Take five or ten minutes to prepare your we/they lists. Pick the one that seems to cause the most feeling. Write down ideas and feelings as specifically as you can. Share this one with your partner(s) and ask them to share their own patterns and experiences around their we/they.

For this exercise, you may want to use only one we/they (i.e. we have diabetes, they don't). But you may be helped more by finding specific distinctions to draw around diet, exercise, control and so on. Repeat the exercise with the 'positives.'

C / Compensations: Alone

Another prominent facet of our participants' experience was their feeling that they had discovered compensations for their perceived limitations. You will recall the reverence for and appreciation of life that was described. Tim recognized that the struggle with diabetes had brought him a sense of accomplishment and self-confidence.

Reflect for a few moments and then quickly list limitations or inadequacies you have because of diabetes (or for other reasons for that matter). Here are a few sentences to complete:
- If I didn't get so worked up ...
- If I had enough money ...
- If I had a better job ...
- If only I could eat anything ...
- When I play too hard ...
- I'm too weak/short/active (or opposites) ...
- I'm too old/immature/slow (or opposites) ...
You can readily extend the list.

Across the page from each of your limitations, write the

compensations you have made. For example, people who were interviewed gave these:
- I have learned to take one day at a time ...
- I'm thankful for each day I get through ...
- I eat candy when I play hockey ...
- My value for life is heightened ...
- Diabetes has made me a stronger person ...

These limitations and compensations may seem too general. Try to identify your own and see how you are making your life work. Try not to judge yourself. If you find some cases where you are not compensating well, try to see how you can handle them differently. This exercise gives you a chance to take stock, get to know yourself better, and to improve your way of handling your diabetes and your life.

D / Compensations: With others

Once again this makes an excellent group exercise, particularly with others who have diabetes.

List your limitations and compensations in three or four categories (physical, diet, feelings, personality, etc.) Select two and talk about them to a partner or to a group. Ask each other person to respond with their experiences so you will have more information to work with. Others may have similar limitations and deal with them much differently. Don't try to change people or even their own approaches. Just give them another point of view.

E / Three portraits

By now you have explored several facets of yourself and your reactions to having diabetes. This exercise may help you pull some of the threads together and think about the future.

Take three pages. On one write 'I WAS,' on the second 'I

AM,' and on the third 'I SHALL BE.' On the top half of each page jot down words, symbols, or pictures to describe yourself in each stage of your life with diabetes. For the future let yourself fantasize freely.

On the bottom half of each page list your reactions, feelings, and any connections between these notes and those on your other pages. What have you missed? Which part has the most information?

Now take three fresh pages and write a one-page portrait of yourself as you were in the past, as you are now, and as you intend to be in the future. You have now reached the end of the exercises. The exercises were all designed to encourage you to reflect upon your life and the place of diabetes in it. You may have found reflection difficult. Don't be discouraged. It is a skill we can learn and the more we do it the better we get. Feel free to return to exercises you have already completed and try them again. You'll probably get new insights. Keep your notes and go back periodically and redo some of the exercises. They will remind you how you have changed and may give you a renewed sense of motivation and direction. Good luck!

Resources for diabetes management

Provincial divisions of Canadian Diabetes Association

British Columbia Division
1091 West 8th Avenue
Vancouver, BC
V6H 1C3

Alberta Division
McCloud Building
Suites 205 & 209
10136-100th Street
Edmonton, Alberta
T5J 0P1

New Brunswick Division
259 Brunswick Street
Fredricton, NB
E3B 1G8

Nova Scotia Division
1221 Barrington Street
Halifax, NS
B3J 1Y2

Manitoba Divison
173 McDermot Avenue
Winnipeg, Manitoba
R3B 0S1

Saskatchewan & District
305 Central Chambers
219-22nd Street East
Saskatoon, Saskatchewan
S7K 0G4

Ontario Division
P.O. Box 2603
London, Ontario
N6A 4C9

Newfoundland Division
P.O. Box 9130
St. John's, Nfld.
A1A 2Y3

Prince Edward Island Division
Box 133
Charlottetown, PEI
C1A 7K2

Quebec Diabetes Association

L'Association du Diabète du Québec
1114, rue Saint Dominique
Montreal, Québec
H2X 3V6

Literature from the Canadian Diabetes Association

The following materials are available free of charge:

Nutritional literature

Alcohol and Diabetes – Do They Mix?
Birthday Bonanza
Eating Out
Metric Measures
The Diabetic Way of Eating
Nutritional Considerations in Diabetes and Pregnancy
Diabetes over 60 – Meals to Serve You Well   (Eng/Fr)
Planning Meals for Your Diabetic Guest
Example Eating Plans and Menus
Diabetic Foods – A Common Sense Approach

Educational literature

Just Like Any Other Kid
Your Eyes and Teeth Matter Too!
Treat Your Feet ... with Care
Diabetes and Pregnancy

The Diabetic's Guide to Health Care
Travelling with Diabetes
Diabetes and Insulin Pumps
Research Horizons
Diabetes and Seniors   (Eng/Fr)
Sync – Getting It All Together   (Eng/Fr)
What about Driving, Dating, Drinking ... and Diabetes?
A Winning Run Is Scored over Diabetes   (Eng/Fr)
Exercise and Diabetes
The Other Side of Diabetes
Pills for Treating Diabetes
Aiming for Good Control in Diabetes
How to Cope with a Brief Illness
Understanding the Complications of Diabetes Mellitus

La littérature française

Sync – votre style de vie
L'etudiant diabètique
Les premiers soins aux diabètiques: Renseignements pour le
   personnel des services des secours
Le diabète et les gens agés
Le diabète après soixante ans: Idées de bons repas
Le diabète mord la poussière
Que faire en cas de maladie de courte durée

Pamphlets

What Is the Canadian Diabetes Association?
What Is Diabetes?

The following materials are available at costs ranging from 60
cents to $13.00 (for the cookbooks)

Nutritional literature

Good Health Eating Guide:

Poster: Good Health Eating Guide
            Vive la santé! Vive la bonne alimentation!
Book: Good Health Eating Guide
            Vive la santé! Vive la bonne alimentation!
Pamphlet: Good Health Eating Guide
            Vive la Santé!Vive la bonne alimentation!

Cookbooks

Light and Easy Choices
Choice Cooking (Eng)
Bien manger = Bonne santé (Fr)
Food Choices in the Market Place

Exchange lists

Meal Planning for Diabetics in Canada, in English – Large
    print only, Italian and Ukrainian
Basic Facts about Your Diabetic Diet (Bilingual Chinese/
    English – simplified version)
Diabetes and Chinese Food (Chinese/English)

Educational literature

Diabetes – A Manual for Canadians
What You Should Know about Pregnancy and Diabetes
Poster: The ups and Downs of Blood Sugar

Non-medical books on diabetes

The following books will provide you with more
information on diabetes:

How to Live with Diabetes, Henry Dolger, MD, and
    Bernard Seeman, 1976, Pyramid Publications, 183 pages

Diabetes without Fear, Dr Joseph I. Goodman, 1978, Avon
Books (Arbor House Publishing Co), 141 pages
The Diabetic's Book, June Biermann and Barbara Toohey,
1981, J.P. Tarcher, Los Angeles, 207 pages
Diabetes, Terri Kivelowitz with Laura Berenson, 1981,
Spectrum – Prentice-Hall, 146 pages
Borrowing Time, Pat Covelli, 1979, Thomas Y. Crowell,
160 pages
Diabetes, James W. Anderson, MD, 1981, Prentice-Hall of
Canada, 157 pages
The Diabetics' Get Fit Book, Jacki Winter, 1984, New
Canada Publications/NC Press, 103 pages
The Diabetic Child, Dr Mimi M. Belmonte, 1983, Eden
Press, 251 pages
Children with Diabetes, Margaret McGill/Robert Vines,
1983, Royal Alexandra Hospital for Children, New
South Wales, 108 pages
Journey of a Diabetic, Lawrence M. Pray with Richard
Evans III, MD, 1983, Simon and Schuster, 202 pages
The Diabetic's Sports and Exercise Book, June Biermann
and Barbara Toohey, 1977, J.B. Lippincott Co, 201 pages
The Peripatetic Diabetic, Margaret Bennett, 1969,
Hawthorn Books, 326 pages
Help Yourself to Health, Ada P. Kahn, MPH, 1983,
Contemporary Books, 121 pages
Take Charge of Your Diabetes, Charles M. Peterson, MD,
1979, Charles M. Peterson, 89 pages
The ABC of Diabetes, Caryl Dow Jorgensen, RN, and John
E. Lewis, PH D, 1979, Crown Publishers, 276 pages
Learning to Live WELL with Diabetes, Donnel D. Etzwiler,
MD, Priscilla Hollander, MD, Marion J. Franz, RD, MS,
Judy Ostrom Joynes RN, MA, 1985, The Diabetes Centre,
Park Nicollet Medical Foundation, Minneapolis,
Minnesota, 382 pages

Children Have Diabetes Too, Staff of Juvenile Diabetes
Clinic of Alberta Children's Hospital, Calgary, Alberta,
1984, 121 pages
You Can't Catch Diabetes from a Friend, Lynne Kipnis and
Susan Adler, 1979, Triad Publishing Co., 64 pages
The Physician Within: Taking Charge of Your Well-Being,
Catherine Feste, 1987, Diabetes Centre, Wayzata,
Minnesota, 169 pages
Diabetes. A Beyond Basics Guide, Rowan Hillson, 1987,
Prentice-Hall Canada, 143 pages

Self-Help Literature

**Developing Support Groups: A Manual for Facilitators and
Participants**, Howard Kirschenbaum and Barbara Glazer,
1978, University Associates, 80 pages
From Self-Help to Health: A Guide to Self-Help Groups,
David Robinson and Yvonne Robinson, 1979, David and
Charles
**Helping You Helps Me: A Guide Book for Self-Help
Groups**, K. Hill, 1984, Canadian Council on Social
Development